SMARTER RECOVERY

A Practical Guide to Maximizing Training Results

Pete McCall, CSCS

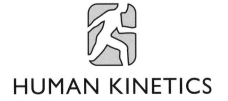

HUMAN KINETICS

Library of Congress Cataloging-in-Publication Data

Names: McCall, Pete, 1972- author.

Title: Smarter recovery : a practical guide to maximizing training results / Pete McCall, CSCS.

Description: Champaign, IL : Human Kinetics, [2024] | Includes bibliographical references and index.

Identifiers: LCCN 2023014562 (print) | LCCN 2023014563 (ebook) | ISBN 9781718214811 (paperback) | ISBN 9781718214828 (epub) | ISBN 9781718214835 (pdf)

Subjects: LCSH: Exercise--Physiological aspects. | Sports--Physiological aspects. | Stress (Physiology) | BISAC: HEALTH & FITNESS / Exercise / General | HEALTH & FITNESS / Massage & Reflexology

Classification: LCC RC1235 .M37 2024 (print) | LCC RC1235 (ebook) | DDC 613.7/1--dc23/eng/20230527

LC record available at https://lccn.loc.gov/2023014562

LC ebook record available at https://lccn.loc.gov/2023014563

ISBN: 978-1-7182-1481-1 (print)

This publication is written and published to provide accurate and authoritative information relevant to the subject matter presented. It is published and sold with the understanding that the author and publisher are not engaged in rendering legal, medical, or other professional services by reason of their authorship or publication of this work. If medical or other expert assistance is required, the services of a competent professional person should be sought.

The web addresses cited in this text were current as of February 2023, unless otherwise noted.

Senior Acquisitions Editor: Michelle Earle; **Developmental Editor:** Anne Hall; **Managing Editor:** Hannah Werner; **Copyeditor:** Jenny MacKay; **Indexer:** Andrea J. Hepner; **Permissions Manager:** Laurel Mitchell; **Senior Graphic Designer:** Sean Roosevelt; **Cover Designer:** Keri Evans; **Cover Design Specialist:** Susan Rothermel Allen; **Photograph (cover):** Georgiy Datsenko/iStock/Getty Images; **Photographs (interior):** Graham Koffler, photos in chapters 5 and 7; All other photos © Human Kinetics, unless otherwise noted; **Photo Asset Manager:** Laura Fitch; **Photo Production Manager:** Jason Allen; **Senior Art Manager:** Kelly Hendren; **Illustrations:** © Human Kinetics, unless otherwise noted; **Printer:** Versa Press

We thank Core Health & Fitness in Lake Forest, California, for assistance in providing the location for the photo shoot for this book.

Human Kinetics books are available at special discounts for bulk purchase. Special editions or book excerpts can also be created to specification. For details, contact the Special Sales Manager at Human Kinetics.

Printed in the United States of America   10 9 8 7 6 5 4 3 2 1

The paper in this book is certified under a sustainable forestry program.

Human Kinetics
1607 N. Market Street
Champaign, IL 61820
USA

United States and International
Website: **US.HumanKinetics.com**
Email: info@hkusa.com
Phone: 1-800-747-4457

Canada
Website: **Canada.HumanKinetics.com**
Email: info@hkcanada.com

E8730

SMARTER RECOVERY

A Practical Guide to Maximizing Training Results

CONTENTS

PART I Recovery Explained   1

1 Understanding the Need for Recovery   3

Learn how your body responds to different exercise demands.
Use the information in this chapter to make recovery an integral
part of every workout to maximize your fitness goals.

2 Impact of Intensity   19

Understand the connection between exercise intensity
and the body's need for repair so you can monitor intensity
to allow for adequate recovery.

3 Systems Overload   35

Optimize your body's natural recovery mechanisms and understand
their response to stress on various internal systems.

4 Recovery Methods   47

Choose the type of recovery method that works best
for your body, your workouts, and your budget.

5 Fascia and Foam Rolling   57

Explore the functions of fascia and the science behind maintaining
healthy muscle development through tissue treatment.

v

EXERCISE FINDER

ACKNOWLEDGMENTS

A book is not created by a single individual. Rather, it takes an entire team to bring a concept to life. First, to all the team members at Human Kinetics, thank you for your tireless efforts to make this book happen. To my clients and group fitness participants, thank you for trusting me with your bodies, and thank you for inspiring me to learn as much about fitness as possible. To my colleagues and teammates, thank you for setting the pace and driving me to try to get one-percent better every day. Finally, to my family—Monica, Parker, Ryan, my parents, David, Bill, and Barbara—thank you for everything, especially your love and support.

INTRODUCTION

For years, the purpose of exercise science was to understand how to help athletes improve performance for a particular sport. From Scandinavian researchers who developed the concept of interval training to sport scientists in the Soviet Union who identified the benefits of periodization, research on exercise was driven by the question of how to help athletes perform better in their specific sport or activity. Understanding how exercise can help people run faster, jump higher, lift more weight, and throw farther is important. However, that is only one part of the equation. Exercise is physical stress imposed on the physiological systems of the body. Scientists have spent most of their time studying the performance outcomes of exercise. However, while doing the work is essential, exercise is only the *process* of applying the stress. It is the time *after* exercise when the various systems of the body adapt to the work performed. Only during the past decade or so have scientists developed a better understanding of how the body recovers from exercise—and more importantly, how these findings can help human performance. The research on recovery is remarkable; it is allowing scientists to identify various strategies and techniques athletes can apply to return the body to homeostasis, the technical term for the normal operating condition of the human body, once a workout is over, which helps them improve their performance. (A strategy is a general approach, such as rehydrating within a short time frame after exercise. A technique is a specific action that applies a strategy, such as drinking a glucose-based sport beverage after exercise to help the body rehydrate faster.)

Performance Training in the Gym

I earned my first personal trainer certification in 1998, from the American Council on Exercise (ACE). (Ten years later, I went to work for the organization.) As I was developing exercise programs for clients and teaching group fitness classes, I would study how athletes exercised and apply that knowledge to the workouts I was designing for both individuals and groups. Since the early days of my career, my belief has been that if a particular technique could help an athlete succeed in competition, it could help my clients reach their own personal fitness goals. My clients and group fitness participants understood that they were exercising the same way elite athletes train—to improve performance. If something worked for an individual who was paid to play a game, then it could work for them as well.

Here is a startling revelation: Until the late 1970s and early 1980s, sport coaches in the United States did not want their athletes lifting weights. The belief was that having too much muscle could actually impede athletic performance. This explains the origins of spring training for professional baseball teams and summer training camps for football teams; after a couple of months away from their sport, athletes needed to play their way back into shape to prepare for the season. If there was no specific, mindful approach to exercise in preparation for competition, then it stands to reason there was no thought given to what athletes should be doing immediately after one competition to prepare for the next. If athletes followed any specific protocol after a training session or game, it was most likely to eat a meal, maybe have a cocktail to unwind (or four, if it was after a game), and enjoy the social scene in whatever city they happened to be in.

Recovery From Exercise

A common definition of the word *recovery* is the process of overcoming an addiction. However, due to an extensive body of research combined with numerous examples of athletes setting new records, the word now has a second meaning in sport vernacular: resting in order to let the body adapt to the physical work performed during exercise. Thanks to elite athletes such as Tom Brady, Drew Brees, and LeBron James, who have managed to sustain or even improve their performance as the years have passed, we have a much better understanding of the role that rest and recovery play in the efforts on a field or court. (I would like to buy each of them a kale smoothie, because they have made my work as a fitness professional and educator so much easier by providing examples of how a systematic approach to recovery can boost performance.)

The field of sport science is focused on how to improve performance. In the early 20th century, Scandinavian coaches observed that shorter, more intense bursts of running followed by brief periods of rest could improve aerobic capacity more efficiently than simply running to the point of exhaustion. In the 1960s, sport scientists in the Soviet Union learned that designing conditioning programs around planned periods of lower-intensity exercise or rest could help athletes perform their best when it came time to compete in their sport. (As a side note, it was also scientists in the Soviet Union who observed that high-intensity exercise elevates levels of muscle-building hormones such as testosterone, so in addition to the workout programs used to prepare for competition, they established the practice of giving athletes supplemental hormones to help muscles recover more quickly. This led to the arms race for performance-enhancing drugs.)

As sport scientists and conditioning coaches have learned, when it comes to elevating human performance, what is done *after* exercise or competition is almost as important as what is done *during* exercise. Now, in the third decade of the 21st century, specific protocols have been established for what to do after one workout or game (or match or meet) to prepare for the next. For example, once athletes have completed a tough conditioning workout or competition, they will most likely have a smoothie, snack, or meal created by a registered dietitian-nutritionist for specific nutritional needs; perform tissue treatment by using a foam roller or percussion gun or receiving a massage; sit in a cryo chamber at −300 degrees Fahrenheit (−184 degrees Celsius), in a hot tub, or in an infrared sauna to help improve circulation; and try to get at least eight hours of uninterrupted sleep, either wearing special garments or on special sheets that have been engineered to help the body recover from stress. Just like sport scientists have established the benefits of year-round conditioning for athletes, there is now a much better understanding of how to help the body recover from one workout so it can be fully prepared for the next.

Applying the Information

When it comes to workouts performed by mainstream fitness enthusiasts, a common belief is that every workout should be extremely challenging, yet nothing could be further from the truth. As you are about to learn, when you have specific fitness goals, exercise is only part of the equation for your workouts to produce the results you want. What you do after you train or compete can speed up the recovery process, allowing you to train at a higher volume, and *that* is what can help you improve your performance. Understanding how working out affects your body, and specifically, how the various physiological systems adapt to the exercises you do in your workouts, could help you identify the most effective strategies for reaching your goals. A mindful approach to recovery can help reduce the risk of injury while maximizing the results you are working for.

Recovery is important after high-intensity workouts. High-intensity exercise was once used mostly by athletes preparing for a sport. However, because it can produce the results many fitness enthusiasts want, such as losing excess body fat or increasing lean muscle mass, in the 2000s, it became an established component of the mainstream fitness culture. While high-intensity exercise itself is not dangerous, too much of it could result in overtraining syndrome. Overtraining occurs when not enough time is allowed for the body to adapt to exercise and could result in a number of negative outcomes, from lingering injuries to illness and depression, that could keep you from achieving the results you want from your workouts.

The Focus of My Career

In 2008, I went to work for ACE to develop education programs for fitness professionals. ACE offers four certification programs: Personal Trainer, Group Fitness Instructor, Health Coach, and Medical Exercise Specialist. Each certification requires professionals to complete 20 hours of continuing education every two years to maintain their credential. My job at ACE was to design and teach these continuing education programs. Around 2010, when the trend of high-intensity workouts was still growing, I realized the need to educate ACE-certified fitness professionals on the role of recovery in exercise-program design. There is nothing wrong with high-intensity exercise if it is done in an appropriate manner; however, much of the time, it is not. As a result, I began studying, teaching, and writing about the science of recovery to help fitness professionals understand that although high-intensity exercise can produce tremendous gains, without the proper postworkout recovery, there is serious risk of overtraining, which can impede results.

For years, I have studied the role of recovery in exercise. My two previous books, *Smarter Workouts: The Science of Exercise Made Simple* and *Ageless Intensity: High-Intensity Workouts to Slow the Aging Process*, both discuss how to apply the science of interval training and periodization to design workout programs that optimize recovery. The science of recovery continues to evolve, and athletes are now able to implement strategies that can help them remain competitive for years longer. Some of these techniques may be expensive, but many are available for reasonable prices. You may not be able to afford a personal chef or registered dietitian-nutritionist, but with some planning and preparation, you most certainly can plan and prepare meals that will help replace energy after a hard training session or competition. And while employing a personal massage therapist may not be in your budget, you can use a foam roller or percussion gun to promote recovery in your muscles and connective tissues. To help you learn how to apply the information, this book features narratives of four different individuals, discussing how each person uses recovery strategies in his or her specific situation.

More than 20 years into my fitness career, I still firmly believe that if a specific technique is good enough for a professional athlete, it is one you should consider using in your own workout program. Why let only elite and professional athletes reap the benefits of the science behind how the body recovers from exercise? This book was written to provide an overview of the existing research on the science of exercise recovery and identify a variety of specific strategies and techniques that can help you experience optimal results from your workout program. Keep in mind that research is constantly evolving, and there may be future findings that dispute those referenced here. Learning the science—and, more importantly, how to apply it—will help.

High-intensity exercise yields many benefits, but to optimize the results from your training program, it is a good idea to recover as hard as you exercise. In short: Train hard, recover harder.

PART I

RECOVERY EXPLAINED

1

UNDERSTANDING THE NEED FOR RECOVERY

Does this sound familiar?

You absolutely love to exercise, push yourself, and sweat hard, and you appreciate the exhaustion that comes from a high-intensity workout. However, you don't always get the results you want, because after a few days of hard workouts, you feel like your battery is drained and you just don't have the energy to succeed.

Whether you are training to achieve success in a specific sport or recreational activity, are working toward a particular fitness goal, or are an instructor responsible for teaching exercise to others, it can be easy to get carried away with exercise, because if a little is good for you, shouldn't more be better? Unfortunately, that is not always the case. Exercise is physical stress imposed on the body. When the body is stressed consistently without appropriate time to allow physiological systems to rest and recover, it could eventually result in overtraining syndrome (OTS). Bandyopadhyay, Bhattacharjee, and Sousana (2012, 7) describe OTS as "the result of an imbalance between stress and recovery. It is a physical, behavioural and emotional condition that occurs when the volume and intensity of an individual's exercise surpasses their recuperation capacity. The progress of athletic performance is ceased, and can even lead to a drop in strength and fitness."

Exercise optimizes your genetic potential. It can help you add lean muscle mass to move faster or lift more weight. It can also enhance aerobic capacity to improve your overall endurance and extend the time it takes to reach muscle fatigue. Another important benefit from elevating your aerobic capacity is being able to recover more quickly from high-intensity bouts during a workout or once the exercise session (or competition) is over. High-intensity exercise, both strength training and metabolic conditioning, can be the most effective and efficient method for making these changes. However, if high-intensity exercise is performed too often without appropriate rest, rehydration, and refueling between exercise sessions, OTS can occur.

Recovery Strategies Enhance Performance

Once upon a time, little thought was given to what should be done after a workout or competition. After a game or hard practice, an athlete might ice a strained muscle or sit in a hot tub, but the general routine was shower, change, get something to eat, and maybe enjoy a few adult beverages. Professional and elite amateur athletes have learned that taking a specific approach to the postworkout recovery process can reduce the time it takes to be ready for the next grueling training session or competition. Here's some great news: The same recovery strategies that help top professional athletes perform at the highest levels of a particular sport could also help you reach your goals with a low risk of injury and reduce overall stress in your life.

A recent phenomenon—the concept of load management—has taken root in the National Basketball Association (NBA). During the competitive season, which runs from October through April, NBA teams play 82 games and often play three times a week, sometimes in multiple cities. The training, competition, and travel schedule for NBA players places tremendous physical demand on the athletes during the six-and-a-half–month season, and they have extremely limited time to rest before the next workout or game. As a result, some players have begun to sit out of games against less competitive teams so they can be fully rested prior to the next game against a challenging opponent. The concept of resting players who are not injured has created some controversy in professional sports. On one hand, athletes are paid extraordinary sums of money for their skills; if the schedule is too exhausting, it could result in poor performance at best and a debilitating injury at worst, making rest essential so a team can protect its investment of a player's salary. On the other hand, fans pay to see the games, and if a star player isn't on the floor, they may feel cheated.

The Role of Recovery

This chapter will help you understand what recovery is and, more importantly, the role it should play in your exercise program. You may not compete as a professional athlete, but your ability to recover completely and effectively affects your training and how you feel before your next workout just as much. The following chapters will identify various strategies and techniques you can use to promote recovery and will explain how and when to apply them so they have the greatest effect on you and your workouts. Keep in mind that the published research can provide insights into physiological processes and explain how a particular method of recovery works, but when it comes to finding specific techniques to meet your needs, it may take some trial and error to identify the most effective ones.

It could be argued that professional athletes deserve their extraordinary salaries because they must always be prepared to compete and win at the highest level of their chosen sport. The high-intensity workouts required to prepare for competition, combined with the physical demands of the games themselves, can place tremendous stress on the physiological systems of the body. There has been a notable increase in research on the topic of postexercise recovery, which allows teams to identify the most effective techniques for helping athletes recover quickly after strenuous physical activity. Professional athletes exercise and compete at the highest levels of intensity, and the teams that help their athletes recover quickly from the demands of one competition so they can be completely rested by the next have an important advantage against their opponents.

Conditioning coaches who work with elite athletes know a secret that many exercise enthusiasts overlook: The most important part of any workout actually occurs *after* the exercise itself. It isn't necessarily the specific exercises used in an athlete's workout that are most important; it's how the overall program is structured to allow time for optimal rest and recovery between training sessions and competitions. Conditioning coaches apply the latest research to help their athletes accelerate the recovery process so they can be completely prepared to deliver an optimal performance.

Professional athletes spend time physically preparing for their sport, but because their bodies are the means for generating an income, they also invest significant money in postexercise recovery strategies to help ensure they can achieve optimal performance. NBA legend LeBron James is known for spending upward of one million dollars per year on various nutrition and recovery strategies so that he can perform his best during every game.

The Purpose of Exercise

Exercise disrupts homeostasis. The recovery process is the complete return to homeostasis and is when muscles and physiological systems adapt to the exercise performed during the workout. Whether you want to add muscle mass or increase energy expenditure to get rid of body fat, disrupting homeostasis by exercising to a point of fatigue (the inability to perform another repetition of an exercise) can be the most effective means of making the desired changes to your body. Fatigue indicates that muscles have used all available energy and require a rest period to replenish energy stores so exercise can continue. It's the period *after* exercise, as the body returns to homeostasis, when muscles adapt and grow, especially after they have worked to the point of fatigue. Moderate- to high-intensity exercise is good for you; however, too many workouts in a row or not allowing the appropriate time for muscles to fully recover after reaching a point of fatigue could result in OTS.

Exercise to the point of fatigue is good for your body and can provide numerous health benefits. The *Physical Activity Guidelines for Americans* published by the United States Department of Health and Human Services state that 150 to 300 minutes a week of moderate-intensity exercise, 75 to 150 minutes a week of vigorous-intensity exercise, or a combination of the two is required to achieve optimal health (Department of Health and Human Services 2018). However, too many workouts to the point of fatigue could result in a cascading accumulation of health issues classified as symptoms of OTS.

When Fatigue Becomes a Bad Thing

To change your body, exercise should be performed to a point of fatigue, but exercising at that level of intensity more than four times per week may not allow enough time between workouts for optimal muscle recovery. Doing too many high-intensity workouts in a row without proper time to fully recover and refuel can result in acute fatigue, the initial phase of overtraining.

Overtraining syndrome is an accumulation of stress and fatigue that occurs as a result of repeatedly exercising to the point of physical exhaustion without allowing adequate time between training sessions to completely rest, repair, rehydrate, and refuel. Overtraining syndrome can be difficult to identify because there is no individual marker; rather, it is an accumulation of various stressors. For example, localized muscle fatigue occurs at the end of a set of repetitions when the muscle cells are rapidly depleted of the energy to fuel contractions. The fatigue usually dissipates, and the muscle can generate force again after a brief rest interval. On the other hand, when not enough rest is allowed between challenging workouts, overall fatigue can affect your entire body and leave you incapable of maintaining your normal level of physical activity. If you feel stale or tired and cannot improve your running times or add weight to your lifts, or if you lie in bed at night unable to fall asleep even though you are exhausted, you may be experiencing overall fatigue, which could evolve into OTS if not addressed with appropriate recovery strategies.

It is important to recognize fatigue when it occurs so you can adapt your exercise routine to overcome it and fully return to homeostasis. Bodybuilders know that exercise to the point of fatigue is the most effective means of enhancing muscle growth and definition, but they use split routines that focus on only one muscle group, which is then allowed to recover (and grow) during the next workout while other muscles are being used. As a different example, strength and conditioning coaches design workout programs for athletes that feature variable levels of intensity to initiate the desired adaptations but allow time to completely recover before a competition. Whether your goals are for physique or performance, the approach to making adaptations and achieving the results you want should be the same: Exercise to the point of momentary muscle fatigue that does not let you perform another repetition, allow an appropriate recovery period, and repeat.

Different Types of Fatigue

Overtraining syndrome is an accumulation of stress that is left untreated, resulting in overall fatigue. Every workout should apply an appropriate training overload to stimulate the desired physical adaptations; however, once the workout is over, specific strategies can help facilitate the return to homeostasis, allowing for a more effective recovery process. Knowing that fatigue could lead to OTS should motivate you to properly monitor and record the intensity, volume, and duration of your workouts and identify the proper amount of rest for the amount of exercise you are doing. Recording the amount of exercise you perform, along with how you feel in terms of overall exhaustion and mindset once the workout is over, can help you identify the onset of fatigue and the need for specific recovery interventions.

Overtraining syndrome starts with acute muscle fatigue, which often occurs after strenuous exercise and is indicated by delayed-onset muscle soreness (DOMS). This can accumulate until multiple symptoms of OTS are present and performance becomes inhibited. The stages of accumulated stress that result in OTS are identified in the following sections.

Acute Fatigue

Acute fatigue can be defined as a short-term, acute response that occurs during intense exercise or competition. Reaching a point of fatigue means that muscle cells have used all the available energy and there is an accumulation of by-products, primarily from anaerobic metabolism, that could disrupt a muscle's ability to contract effectively. Fatigue indicates that muscles need time, either between sets or after a workout, to rest, rehydrate, repair, and recover. In the short term, fatigue is a good thing; it means the muscles have worked hard enough to stimulate desired changes. During the course of an exercise program, however, too many workouts to the point of fatigue without proper recovery after each one could result in OTS and keep you from achieving your desired outcomes.

An accumulation of acute fatigue could cause two specific types of chronic fatigue: peripheral or central.

Peripheral Fatigue

Peripheral fatigue is the feeling that muscles are out of gas and cannot function at normal levels. It is the effect of a biochemical and metabolic response that occurs in muscle cells as the result of depleting available energy stores; it can impair muscle function and is associated with the volume and intensity of exercise. Cramping, which can occur as a result of dehydration combined with a loss of electrolytes, is an indication of peripheral fatigue. Proper nutrition is required to replace energy and promote tissue repair before muscles can perform at high exertion again.

Central Fatigue

Central fatigue affects the central nervous system—specifically, the ability of motor neurons to synapse effectively with their attached muscle fibers—and is a result of fluctuating levels of calcium (an electrolyte) and acetylcholine (a neurotransmitter) that influence a muscle's ability to contract (Kenney, Wilmore, and Costill 2022). If you have ever been so exhausted that your arms and legs felt like they weighed hundreds of pounds, or if a workout was so fatiguing that you felt like you were moving in slow motion at the end, you have most likely experienced central fatigue.

A single workout or competition could result in acute fatigue, which is addressed with proper postexercise nutrition and rest, specifically sleep. Inadequate sleep or a lack of proper nutrition could result in an accumulation of fatigue that leads to either central or peripheral fatigue and keeps you from achieving an optimal level of performance.

Delayed-Onset Muscle Soreness

Everyone has done it. You return to the gym after a few weeks (or years) of not exercising and do what feels like a "normal" workout only to wake up incredibly sore the next day, to the point where every movement seems to create new levels of discomfort. This is an indication of delayed-onset muscle soreness (DOMS), which is caused by extremely high levels of tension in the contractile element of muscle fibers during exercise. While not fatal, DOMS is certainly uncomfortable. You may have experienced it and wondered how exercise, which is supposed to be good for you, could cause so much discomfort, but DOMS is actually part of the healing process.

Exercise to the point of fatigue creates both mechanical and metabolic overload, which, in turn, could result in DOMS. Applying an appropriate amount of overload to initiate changes should leave muscles a little sore the next day, an indication that they have worked beyond their existing capacity. Although a little soreness is appropriate, exercise should not result in extreme discomfort. Repeated muscle contractions producing high force can cause structural damage to cell membranes and the connective tissues that surround individual muscle fibers (Kenney, Wilmore, and Costill 2022). The following list explains how the body copes with such damage:

- Damage to cell membranes changes calcium levels in the involved muscle fibers; this inhibits cellular respiration, the process of producing energy. High calcium concentrations can activate enzymes that impede the ability of muscle fibers to contract.

Functional Overreach

Exercise can help athletes optimize their genetic potential for their chosen sport, and a functional overreach uses high-intensity exercise to the point of fatigue as an effective means of achieving that outcome. Functional overreaching refers to performing a series of high-intensity workouts in a brief period, usually less than a week, followed by a few days of planned rest before the start of an athletic event or competitive season. The purpose of functional overreaching is to condition physiological systems to become more efficient at working through fatigue—specifically, metabolizing the energy required for muscle contractions. The goal of a planned period of overexertion is to disrupt homeostasis by overstressing the body with a series of challenging workouts or training sessions before allowing time for muscles to rest and completely recover before the competition. If you have ever followed a running program that challenged you to gradually increase the distance and intensity of your runs before giving you a few days of rest before the event, you have used functional overreaching.

- A few hours after the structural damage, there is an elevation in the level of neutrophils, immune cells that promote the inflammatory response necessary for tissue repair.
- Macrophage activity and intracellular contents that accumulate outside muscle cells activate the free nerve endings in muscle tissue.
- Fluids and electrolytes move into the damaged area, which can cause swelling that stimulates pain receptors in muscle tissue. Even though the inflammatory process is helping to repair and heal the damaged tissues, the pressure from the swelling causes the discomfort of DOMS.

Delayed-onset muscle soreness could disrupt the ability of muscles to generate force and result in decreased strength. This is the challenge of designing an exercise program: You want to work hard enough to feel the results of the workouts, but you should not be sore to the point where moving is uncomfortable. If you feel that you can exercise a little harder, it is easy to increase the intensity with the next workout; however, if you exercise too much, it could cause DOMS, which will interrupt your ability to train. Delayed-onset muscle soreness is a sign that fatigue has been achieved and is a good indicator that specific recovery strategies should be applied to help reduce the soreness and return to homeostasis.

Case Study: Functional Overreaching in Practice

Sam and Fred are twin brothers who enjoy competing in half and full marathons. The final two weeks before their most recent marathon provides an excellent example of the difference between a functional overreach and overtraining.

The race was on the 15th of the month. Each brother had raced a half marathon six weeks earlier, so they should have each been prepared to do well at this event. For the first seven days of the month, Sam performed a functional overreach. He pushed himself to train hard every day and progressed the intensity of his workouts so that his longest run matched the pace he would try to hold on race day. After the first week, Sam started cutting back on mileage and slowing his pace to reduce the stress on his body. At the same time, he increased his carbohydrate consumption so that he would have more muscle glycogen available during race day. By the 10th of the month, Sam stopped running altogether and spent the remaining five days doing light physical activity and eating a normal diet so that he would be properly rested and well fueled before the event.

On the other hand, Fred's spouse scheduled a vacation for the first week of the month on an island that did not have 26 miles (42 km) of road for him to run on. Fred spent the first week of the month doing what exercise he could, and when he returned home, he resumed his normal running schedule. However, because he had missed crucial training time, Fred maintained his mileage and pace until three days before the race rather than allowing more time for his body to rest. With his experience, Fred thought that three days would be enough recovery time. However, once the race started, Fred's legs felt heavy, and he never felt like he was able to achieve his normal running tempo. As a result, he ran one of the worst races of his career. Sam, in contrast, started the race well rested and full of energy, which allowed him to post a personal record in the marathon.

Sam followed the protocol for an effective functional overreach and experienced the benefits. Fred did not plan his workouts well, and as a result, he started the race in a slightly fatigued state, which limited his performance.

Nonfunctional Overreach

In the short term, overworking muscles for a few workouts in a row can help initiate adaptations; however, too many overreach days in a row with insufficient rest and recovery could result in nonfunctional overreaching, which could easily end up as overtraining. Figure 1.1 demonstrates how physical stress can accumulate and result in overtraining syndrome. The time for complete recovery is indicated for each stage. Multiple challenging, moderate- to high-intensity workouts can deplete available energy sources and cause short-term (acute) fatigue, which is remedied with proper nutrition and sleep. A functional overreach should be designed to mimic the physiological stress experienced during competition; however, a few days of rest and healthy eating before the competition are necessary to help muscles fully replenish energy stores. It is important to keep the rest period relatively brief, because detraining—the loss of strength or aerobic endurance—could occur after as little as two weeks if there is no strenuous physical activity. However, not allowing adequate rest between the end of the overreach phase and the competition could result in poor performance, a clear indicator of nonfunctional overreaching. (Note: Nonfunctional overreaching could also occur as the result of participating in a multiday event such as a tournament or ultra-endurance race; participating in that type of excessive activity requires a planned recovery strategy to effectively return to homeostasis.)

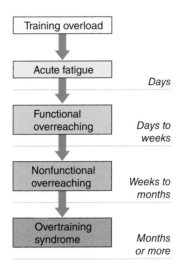

FIGURE 1.1   The overtraining continuum.

How to Identify OTS

Snyder and Hackney (2013, 524) note,

> Unfortunately, little is known about the adaptation process and the recovery needed to maximize physiological adaptations and thus exercise performance. What may work for one athlete may not work for another, as everyone responds to stress in a different manner: one athlete may adapt to a training program, while another may have performance decrements due to overtraining on the same program. The border between training adaptation and performance enhancements and overtraining and performance decrements is not concrete, and probably involves other factors (or stresses) than just exercise training.

Since Snyder and Hackney wrote this in the early 2010s, researchers have been studying how to mitigate the effects of cumulative stress and there is now a much greater understanding of the need for proper rest to allow for adaptations to occur and to prevent overtraining. Inadequate rest between high-intensity exercise sessions or working out too many days in a row are the most likely causes of OTS, which could lead to chronic fatigue, reduced physical performance, mood changes, neuroendocrine system imbalances, and frequent illness. The challenge with identifying the difference between being fatigued from a single workout or overtrained from excessive exercise is that there is not a single physiological marker to indicate OTS. Common symptoms of OTS and their effects are identified in table 1.1.

TABLE 1.1 Symptoms and Effects of Overtraining Syndrome (OTS)

SYMPTOM	EFFECT
Reduced immune system function	Cortisol can suppress the immune system and increase the risk of developing an infection or catching a virus, which can limit the ability to exercise. A lingering cold, upper respiratory tract infection, or other illness that does not seem to go away could be a possible indication of OTS.
Chronic muscle soreness	A challenging workout could result in DOMS, acute muscle soreness lasting 24 to 72 hours. Excessive or lingering muscle soreness that lasts for days after exercise could indicate OTS.
Disruption of the normal sleep cycle, despite feeling physically fatigued	The adrenocortical system, a component of the SNS, regulates the primary neuroendocrine response to exercise by releasing the catabolic hormones and catecholamines responsible for energy production. An imbalance between anabolic and catabolic hormones could affect the ability to fall asleep even when physically fatigued. A lack of sleep impedes recovery, allowing more exercise stress to accumulate.
Elevated resting heart rate	An overstimulated SNS can elevate the resting heart rate. The SNS regulates production of cortisol, epinephrine, and norepinephrine, all of which help provide energy for exercise by elevating the heart rate, dilating blood vessels, and releasing free fatty acids. Excessive SNS activity with inadequate recovery could start with an elevated resting heart rate but ultimately result in adrenal fatigue and a host of health issues.
Cognitive decline that can affect mood, the ability to process information, and decision-making	During sleep, the brain produces proteins that help remove unnecessary plaques and keep neurons functioning optimally. Interrupted sleep patterns could result in a decline in cognitive function. In a study published in the journal *Nature Communications*, researchers observed that adults between the ages of 50 and 70 years who averaged less than 6 hours of sleep per night had a much higher risk of developing cognitive decline or dementia in their later years when compared with those who consistently slept more than 6 hours per night (Sabia et al. 2021).
Weight gain despite regular exercise	Too much exercise without proper nutrition that includes optimal amounts of carbohydrates, fat, or protein could result in weight gain. Gluconeogenesis occurs when protein, as opposed to fat or carbohydrates, is used for fuel; those macronutrients could be stored as free fatty acids in adipose tissue for use at a later date.
Changes to overall mood, increased irritability, and an elevated risk of depression	Lack of sleep and low performance can trigger a cycle of depression and self-doubt about the ability to perform physical activity at a high level. Snyder and Hackney (2013) noted that up to 80% of athletes who experience OTS also report significant mood changes and increased bouts of depression. The central-fatigue hypothesis suggests that because the brain functions to protect muscles from damage as the result of excessive exercise, an accumulation of exercise stress could change the chemistry of the brain. This could have an effect on mood states in athletes (Bishop, Jones, and Woods 2008).
Lower performance in routine training activities	Elevated levels of catabolic hormones could suppress testosterone production and limit the amount available for postexercise protein synthesis and tissue repair (Snyder and Hackney 2013). When sufficient testosterone is not produced to support the necessary postexercise tissue repair, it could change the ability of muscles to recover after exercise and may result in not being able to complete standard training lifts or distances.

Abbreviations: DOMS, delayed-onset muscle soreness; SNS, sympathetic nervous system.

Adapted from Hausswirth and Mujika (2013).

Optimize Your Recovery

Because OTS is the result of excessive exercise combined with inappropriate recovery between exercise sessions, using metrics to track performance of your workouts, combined with taking daily notes about your overall energy, mindset, and fatigue, can be the easiest way to identify when your body is not responding as it should to a workout program. It can be hard to determine whether OTS is caused by too much exercise or a separate health issue. However, monitoring and recording the intensity of your workouts allows you to identify a drop in performance almost immediately and address it with appropriate recovery strategies.

Because there is not a single, specific biological marker indicating overtraining, it can be a challenge to determine when a planned functional overreach has become overtraining or when recovery between high-intensity exercise sessions has been inadequate. In an effort to help coaches identify when OTS occurs, the American College of Sports Medicine and the European College of Sport Science released a joint statement on OTS, describing it as "a long-term decrement in performance capacity with or without related physiological or psychological signs and symptoms of maladaptation in which restoration of performance capacity may take several weeks or months" (Kenney, Wilmore, and Costill 2022, 417). Overtraining syndrome affects the endocrine, neural, metabolic, and immune systems, and it can be difficult to identify its onset using biological markers, because every individual has a different response to exercise and adapts to exercise in his or her own unique way.

Not being able to maintain a consistent pace for a normal training run, lift a typical amount of weight, or perform a routine number of repetitions are all possible indicators that your body needs time to properly recover before it can be relied on to achieve a high level of performance. Keeping consistent, easy-to-read records of your workouts, including your pace, average heart rate, and distance for endurance training or the amount of weight used along with the repetitions and sets completed during strength training sessions, can help identify an accumulation of fatigue, because the only certain sign of OTS is a decrease in performance during competition or training. Table 1.2 lists the various symptoms of anaerobic overtraining; having a system for recording the intensity, quality, and feeling of your workouts allows you to identify when these symptoms start occurring.

TABLE 1.2 Theoretical Development of Anaerobic Overtraining

STAGE OF OVERTRAINING	TIME TO ONSET	PERFORMANCE	NEURAL	SYMPTOMS OF ANAEROBIC PERFORMANCE					
				SKELETAL MUSCLE	METABOLIC	CARDIOVASCULAR	IMMUNE	ENDOCRINE	PSYCHOLOGICAL
Acute fatigue	Days	No effect or increase	Altered neuron function	—	—	—	—	—	—
Functional overreaching	Days to weeks	Temporary decrease; returns to baseline	Altered motor unit recruitment	—	—	—	—	Altered sympathetic activity and hypothalamic control	—
Nonfunctional overreaching	Weeks to months	Stagnation or decrease	Decreased motor coordination	Altered excitation–contraction coupling	Decreased muscle glycogen	Increased resting heart rate and blood pressure	Altered immune function	Altered hormone concentrations	Mood disturbances
Overtraining syndrome	Many months to years	Decrease	—	Decreased force production	Decreased glycolytic capacity	—	Sickness and infection	—	Emotional and sleep disturbances

Reprinted by permission from D. French, "Adaptations to Anaerobic Training Programs," in *NSCA Essentials of Strength Training and Conditioning*, 4th ed., edited for the National Strength and Conditioning Association by G.G. Haff and N.T. Triplett (Champaign, IL: Human Kinetics, 2016); Adapted from A. Fry, *Physiological Responses to Short-Term High Intensity Resistance Exercise Overtraining*, Ph.D. Diss., The Pennsylvania State University (1993); Adapted from Meeusen et al. (2013).

Possible Causes of OTS

Potential contributors to OTS include depletion of available glycogen in muscle cells, exercise-induced tissue damage, inflammation, and oxidative stress (Cheng, Jude, and Lanner 2020). No single component causes OTS; rather, it is an accumulation of physical stress that changes the body's response to exercise. Whether you are a dedicated exercise enthusiast, a weekend warrior, or an elite athlete, when the intensity, duration, and frequency of high-intensity workouts are not carefully monitored, the risk of developing OTS could increase significantly. In the best-case scenario, OTS could result in general fatigue or burnout, culminating in the loss of motivation to exercise or compete. In the worst-case scenario, OTS could result in a debilitating overuse injury such as a ruptured tendon or cause a serious issue such as adrenal fatigue, which could limit the ability to exercise for months at a time.

From a technical standpoint, OTS is a quantifiable loss of performance, which is why it can be much easier to identify in athletes training for competition: They are either improving or they are not. When athletes or their conditioning coach notice they are not improving, it is time to evaluate whether rest or another recovery intervention is necessary. Monitoring and tracking performance during workouts is critical; if you notice you are unable to lift the same amount of weight, complete the same number of repetitions, or maintain the same pace for a specific distance, it could indicate an accumulation of exercise stress, which necessitates a specific recovery strategy. Using quantitative performance metrics to measure exercise intensity, such as monitoring your heart rate or recording the weight and repetitions for each lift, can help you track the amount of work you do and plan the appropriate amount of recovery to reduce the risk of developing OTS.

Metabolic Stress

Exercise to a point of momentary fatigue, the inability to complete another repetition, is the first sign of metabolic stress and an indication that the involved muscle has depleted its available supply of adenosine triphosphate (ATP), the chemical that fuels cellular activity; time is then required to remove the by-products from anaerobic metabolism and produce new ATP to sustain activity. Sport drinks, gels, or gummies contain high amounts of carbohydrates, as well as sodium and other electrolytes, and they provide immediate energy to muscle cells in order to sustain ATP production and delay the onset of fatigue during high-intensity exercise. Immediately after high-intensity exercise is completed, consuming an adequate amount of protein, carbohydrate, and fat is necessary for replacing spent energy, repairing damaged tissue, and supporting other essential physiological functions that help the body return to homeostasis.

Endocrine Response to Exercise

An important goal of many workout programs is to increase the size of muscle tissue and enhance its ability either to rapidly produce force for explosive activities or, for endurance-oriented sports, to sustain force production over an extended time. However, too much exercise can actually impede muscle growth, which is another reason to monitor your workout intensity when you have specific strength- or physique-related goals. As the body is returning to homeostasis after moderate- to high-intensity exercise, the anabolic hormones testosterone, human growth hormone, and insulin-like growth factor 1 are released to support the repair of muscle fibers damaged during exercise. However, excessive exercise or inadequate rest after a hard workout could result in an accumulation of energy-producing hormones, including cortisol and epinephrine, that could interfere with muscle growth. For example, when exercise depletes the amount of available blood glucose, it could result in an accumulation of cortisol, causing gluconeogenesis—the process of converting amino acids, which are normally used to repair damaged muscle proteins, into ATP to provide fuel for muscle contractions. When protein is used for energy during exercise, it can result in less being available to support tissue repair and muscle growth once exercise is over.

Developing a Recovery Mindset

With all the healthy, nutritious foods you can turn into delicious meals, why would you ever limit yourself to a diet of just peanut butter and jelly sandwiches? If you have been doing the same workout program for an extended amount of time, that is essentially what you are doing to your muscles; you are restricting them to a limited diet that could impede their ability to grow. As you will learn in the following chapters, adjusting your workout programs to impose different stimuli on your body and simply making a few adjustments to variables such as repetitions, tempo, and rest intervals could provide the stimulus needed to increase or reduce the overall stress load of a workout.

Some workouts *should* be challenging to produce the desired changes you want to make to your body, but the idea that *all* workouts need to be extremely hard or strenuous is a fallacy. Yes, harder workouts are necessary to stimulate adaptations in your muscles and physiological systems; however, lower-intensity workouts have an important role too as part of the postexercise recovery process to help alleviate discomfort the day after a really hard workout (Hausswirth and Mujika 2013). Instead of pushing yourself to the point of discomfort with every workout, learn how to use lower-intensity exercise to recover from more challenging training sessions or to reduce stress by staying active when your schedule becomes busy. Low- to moderate-intensity mobility workouts can also help reduce muscle tightness and improve blood flow after a long day of limited movement, like being stuck in meetings or sitting in a car or plane. Knowing how to alternate between high- and low-intensity workouts as well as when it might be necessary to exchange a planned high-intensity interval training (HIIT) workout or heavy strength training session for some low-intensity mobility exercises could help you feel better and reduce overall stress levels.

There *is* such a thing as too much exercise. The use of equipment like barbells, kettlebells, or heavy medicine balls for high-intensity strength or power training, combined with the ongoing popularity of HIIT, means that a well-thought-out strategy for recovery is becoming an increasingly crucial component of a workout program. Exercising too hard during a single workout produces temporary soreness, while too many high-intensity workouts in a row without a day or two of rest could result in OTS.

Whether you are an enthusiast who exercises to look better at the beach, a weekend warrior who wants to beat the other people in the ladder at your tennis club, or an athlete working toward a scholarship or professional contract, understanding your recovery needs and how to structure various strategies into your workout program could help you achieve your fitness goals. When it comes to recovery, your mindset should be that tomorrow's workout begins at the end of today's. Hydration to restore fluid levels in muscle and connective tissues, healthy nutrition to replace spent energy, and adequate rest (specifically sleep) are critical during the postworkout recovery process.

An exercise program should be specific to your needs and goals, and a postexercise recovery program is the same. It does not mean just resting on the couch; instead, a recovery program should meet the specific needs of your workouts. The following chapters will go into detail about how specific strategies such as hydration, proper nutrition, elevating circulation, and getting adequate sleep work and when you should use them to help your body heal after a workout. When you know how to apply the most suitable recovery strategies for different workouts, you can train all year long with a lower risk of injury and crush your fitness goals.

2

IMPACT OF INTENSITY

You know the feeling: You're walking through the doors of your gym, you're well fed and feeling well rested, you had a great day at work, and you are ready to get after it during your workout this evening. There is a sense of anticipation for a high-intensity workout that you know will be challenging and leave you drenched in sweat but also feeling great when you're done. Workouts or training sessions that you know will be at a high intensity, or the highest intensity possible, generate a certain feeling of anticipation not caused by exercising at other intensities. Let's face it—even the best yoga class doesn't build the same type of preworkout energy and leave you feeling the same as a kettlebell-based, high-intensity interval training workout. That's because high-intensity exercise creates different chemical reactions that influence your entire body from the cells up, and that level of intensity will directly influence your ability to recover from a workout.

Not All Exercise Needs to Be High Intensity

Exercise, whether working out or playing competitive sports, is the process of applying physical stress that disrupts homeostasis in order to make desired changes to your body. However, not all exercise is the same, and not all workouts require a specific recovery strategy, making it necessary to define the difference between low-, moderate-, and high-intensity exercise. High-intensity exercise is the most effective for changing the body but is also the most stressful and causes the greatest disruption to homeostasis; therefore, it requires a specific postexercise recovery strategy. Low-intensity workouts do not create a significant disruption to homeostasis, so no specific recovery strategies are necessary. Think of it this way: While absolute rest *is* important, there should never be a reason to skip a workout the day after a challenging exercise session or intense competition, because low-intensity exercise is a form of active recovery and could actually promote the complete return to homeostasis.

High-intensity exercise is good for you and can provide many benefits, but too much of it without enough time to allow a full return to homeostasis between workouts could impede performance and result in overtraining. This helps to explain why professional basketball players use the concept of load management; they realize that to perform their best, they require more rest than was being allowed in their competition and travel schedule. There needs to be a balance between physically demanding activity and rest, because doing too much of one at the expense of the other will result in subpar performance. You may not make the same salary as a professional athlete (sorry about that), but you *can* train the same way at the same level of intensity, and after a hard workout or competition, you should definitely apply the same recovery strategies they use in an effort to help you reach your fitness goals.

The Paradox of Intensity

There is a paradox when it comes to the use of intensity during exercise; too little of it and the body won't make the desired adaptations, but too much could result in overtraining and cause an injury. The lack of proper intensity is a common issue experienced by many fitness enthusiasts who become stuck on a plateau where exercise no longer seems to have the desired effect and the body stops making any adaptations. Exercising at the same intensity for too long is the most common way to become stuck on a plateau. For exercise to have the greatest effect and cause the intended adaptations, it is necessary to learn how to use intensity appropriately and be comfortable with the fact that some workouts should be at an intensity high enough to cause discomfort, whereas others should be at a relatively low intensity—just enough to elevate circulation, which could help muscles to completely recover after hard exercise.

The whole point of a mindful, strategic approach to recovery from exercise is that the faster you can return to homeostasis, the more time your muscles have to refuel, rehydrate, and repair before the next workout, practice session, or competition.

Think of high-intensity exercise as like watching videos on your phone: Yes, you can do it, but it drains your battery quickly, meaning you have to recharge more frequently or carry an external power pack so you can charge while you're watching. High-intensity exercise has the same effect on your muscles; too much high-intensity exercise will deplete muscle cells of stored glycogen, and they will require time to completely replenish this essential source of energy. However, your body probably has an adequate reserve of free fatty acids that can supply energy for low-intensity activity, so on the day after a hard workout, while muscle cells are replacing the energy used the day before, it is perfectly feasible to do an easier workout that causes you to sweat a little without creating any noticeable discomfort.

Creating Balance in Your Exercise Program

One observation of modern life seems to be that if a little is good, then more must be better. Advertising might make you think that more is better for pickup trucks, fast food, or bottles of soda, but when it comes to exercise, specifically moderate- to high-intensity exercise, nothing could be further from the truth. Yes, physiological systems must be challenged to work beyond their existing capacity in order to adapt and work more efficiently. However, for exercise to deliver the intended results, these systems must also be allowed time to rest, rehydrate, refuel, and repair. Having a system for monitoring exercise intensity will allow you to identify which workouts need a specific recovery strategy and which do not. More importantly, monitoring the intensity of your workouts allows you to create a balance between training sessions that stimulate adaptations (hard sessions) and those that reduce overall stress in order to allow those adaptations to occur (lower-intensity sessions).

Intensity is one component of overall training volume, which can be described as the product of the intensity, the number of repetitions performed, and the number of sets completed. Intensity refers to (1) the amount of weight used during a resistance training exercise, (2) the level of effort (or velocity) during a running, swimming, or cycling event, or (3) the overall amount of work performed (work itself is the product of force and distance) during a competition. Developing the optimal recovery strategy for your workout program first requires having a system for monitoring the intensity of workouts along with the overall training volume of the program. Measuring and tracking the intensity and volume of your workouts allows you to be prepared with appropriate recovery strategies after the challenging ones.

Exercise Intensity

There are different methods to describe and quantify exercise intensity; however, the rating of perceived exertion (RPE) may be the easiest to use because it is an estimate of how hard you *feel* you are working and is completely subjective based on your personal ability to tolerate discomfort. The RPE is measured using a 1-to-10 scale, where 1 is the lowest level of intensity (the amount of effort it takes to sit on your couch) and 10 is the highest (the amount of effort it takes to flee from a horde of attacking zombies). Although the RPE does not provide specific feedback on your heart rate or calories burned, it can be an effective tool for monitoring your level of exercise intensity based solely on how you feel as the result of the amount of fatigue caused by a particular exercise session. A review of the research literature (Eston 2012) found that using a scale of perceived exertion can be a valid method for determining the amount of intensity expended by athletes when training for their sport. The RPE can be applied to both resistance training and metabolic conditioning workouts: Strength or power training with near-maximal resistance might have an RPE of 8 out of 10, whereas a mobility workout of bodyweight exercises might have an RPE of only 4 to 6 and a high-intensity interval training workout performed to a point of fatigue might have an RPE of 9. The point of using an RPE is that you can create your own personal system for tracking the intensity of your workouts, allowing you to achieve balance in your training program by scheduling lower-intensity workouts that promote optimal recovery from the harder ones.

Intensity for Resistance Training

Progressive overload refers to the fact that in order to create desired physiological adaptations, exercise must be performed at an intensity greater than the body is currently accustomed to performing (Haff and Triplett 2016). For resistance training, an overload is necessary to make muscles stronger and can be achieved by lifting a heavier load, performing a higher number of repetitions to a point of momentary muscle fatigue where it is not possible to complete another repetition, or shortening the rest interval. Intensity for resistance training can be measured as either the amount of weight lifted (expressed as a percentage of the maximum weight that can be lifted in one repetition for that particular exercise) or the number of repetitions able to be completed before reaching fatigue. There is an inverse relationship between intensity and the number of repetitions able to be performed during a resistance training workout: The heavier the weight, the higher the intensity and the fewer repetitions that can be completed. Whether intensity is quantified by the amount of weight or the number of repetitions, for muscles to stimulate the desired neurological and structural adaptations, they should be exercised to the point of fatigue—the inability to complete another repetition. A heavy, high-intensity load requires muscle fibers to pull against one another to generate the force necessary for producing movement, which results in mechanical stress on the involved tissues. Performing repetitions to the point of momentary muscle fatigue will deplete available energy, imposing significant metabolic stress on the involved muscles. This overload, whether a mechanical overload created by the amount of resistance used or a metabolic overload created by the number of repetitions completed, is necessary to stimulate muscle growth. The type of overload imposed during a workout could influence the strategy used for the postexercise recovery phase.

One-Repetition Maximum

Identifying the percentage of the one-repetition maximum (1RM) for a particular lift is one way to measure intensity for resistance training. Textbooks on resistance training or exercise-program design often include an appendix that lists the values for estimated 1RM based on the number of repetitions able to be completed with a certain amount of weight. For example, according to the 1RM conversion chart in Appendix A of *NASM Essentials of Personal Fitness Training*, 7th edition, performing a lift with 200 pounds for six repetitions is the equivalent of a 235-pound 1RM (Sutton 2021). (Note: An Internet search for *one rep maximum conversion chart* should help you find a table you can use.)

Maximum Repetitions

Another way to describe intensity is to identify the maximum number of repetitions that can be performed for a lift with a specific amount of weight. For example, if an individual can bench press 200 pounds for a total of 10 repetitions and is unable to perform another repetition, then 200 is their 10-repetition maximum (10RM). Either method can be used to assign a specific value of intensity for resistance training.

The Role of Metabolic Conditioning

Activities like cycling, swimming, walking, hiking, or exercising on one of the many machines you'll find in a modern fitness facility, including treadmills, elliptical runners, stationary bikes, or stair climbers, help improve cardiorespiratory efficiency, which is the lungs' ability to put oxygen into the bloodstream combined with how efficiently the heart can pump that oxygenated blood around the body. Because these types of exercises help improve the function of the cardiorespiratory system, they are commonly referred to as cardiovascular exercises, or *cardio* for short.

Your cardiorespiratory system is responsible for pumping oxygenated blood to the working muscles and moving deoxygenated blood back to the lungs. However, here is something to consider: *Any* type of physical activity that elevates your heart rate and pumps oxygenated blood to your working muscles could be considered a mode of cardiovascular exercise. In addition, any exercise that increases oxygen consumption could help burn calories, which means that *cardio* is an accurate but incomplete term to describe exercise performed for the purpose of becoming more energy efficient.

Energy is neither created nor destroyed; it is transferred from one state to another. Energy from macronutrients, specifically fats and carbohydrates, consumed in the diet is stored as potential energy in muscle cells, the liver, and adipose tissue so that it can be released as kinetic energy via muscular activity. *Metabolism* refers to the chemical reactions required to convert fats and carbohydrates into the energy used to support the body's physiological functions, including physical activities such as exercise. While the heart *is* working hard during high-intensity exercise, the reality is that the involved muscles are most likely relying on anaerobic metabolism, which does not require oxygen to produce energy.

While all exercise requires muscle cells to metabolize energy to fuel muscle contractions, specific workouts can help your body become more efficient at producing energy. If the purpose of exercise is to increase the ability to sustain a high work rate or delay the time to fatigue, then *metabolic conditioning* is a more appropriate term, because ultimately, muscles are becoming more efficient at metabolizing energy in order to sustain physical activity for longer periods of time. Hereafter, *metabolic conditioning* will be used to refer to exercise for the purpose of improving efficient energy production.

Metabolic Pathways

Metabolic conditioning, or any exercise that elevates your heart rate, delivers a number of well-established health benefits, including enhanced cardiac efficiency (the ability to move blood around the body), increased mitochondrial density, a reduced risk of developing heart disease, and lower levels of cholesterol and excess body fat—all of which can help improve your overall level of fitness (Haff and Triplett 2016). There are three different pathways for how muscle cells metabolize the energy to fuel contractions: immediate, intermediate, and long term. The immediate pathway involves the limited amount of adenosine triphosphate (ATP) stored in muscle cells. When this stored ATP is depleted, which happens very quickly, muscle cells still need energy and must metabolize more ATP, either by using oxygen combined with fat or carbohydrates (aerobic metabolism) or by using carbohydrates that do not require oxygen to be metabolized into ATP (anaerobic metabolism). The other two pathways are discussed in the next section.

Long-Term and Intermediate Energy Pathways

Low-intensity exercise uses the long-term pathway for ATP, which is dominant in type I muscle fibers, where fat and oxygen are metabolized into ATP via aerobic respiration in cell structures called mitochondria. The intermediate pathway is used for moderate to high levels of exercise intensity, when type II muscle fibers metabolize glycogen (the form in which carbohydrates are stored in muscle cells)—first into glucose, then into ATP. Glycolysis, the process of metabolizing glucose into ATP, can happen either aerobically or anaerobically. Aerobic glycolysis is the process of using oxygen to metabolize glucose into ATP and can yield approximately 36 to 39 molecules of ATP per molecule of glucose. Anaerobic glycolysis does not require oxygen for ATP production and can produce two to three molecules of ATP per molecule of glucose. This is what makes high-intensity exercise so energy expensive (that is, it burns a lot of calories); because one molecule of glucose only yields two to three ATP molecules as the result of anaerobic glycolysis, a lot more glycogen is used during the exercise session, and this glycogen must be replaced during the postexercise recovery process.

By-Products of Anaerobic Metabolism

Glycolysis, whether aerobic or anaerobic, results in a rapid accumulation of by-products including hydrogen ions, inorganic phosphates, and lactate, which in turn elevate blood acidity and create the burning sensation that is felt in working muscles during high-intensity exercise and is often associated with fatigue. High-intensity exercise relies primarily on anaerobic glycolysis and could result in a variety of metabolic by-products that cause feelings of soreness or fatigue during activity. Fatigue is the loss of energy during physical activity and can result in poor performance. High-intensity metabolic conditioning workouts that focus on anaerobic glycolysis can improve muscles' ability to produce ATP and to tolerate the accumulation of by-products in order to delay the onset of fatigue and improve performance. Consistent, high-intensity metabolic conditioning can help enhance overall fitness and improve the ability to recover from bouts of high-intensity exercise; this will be covered in more detail in chapter 9.

The Energy Yield of ATP

The amount of ATP produced during exercise is based on whether glycogen must first be converted to glucose. Carbohydrates consumed in the diet are transported through the blood as glucose and stored in the liver and muscle cells as glycogen, which must be converted to glucose before it can be metabolized into ATP One reason why proper nutrition is such an important component of recovery is that one molecule of ATP yields approximately seven calories of energy; this means that during high-intensity exercise activity, when muscles are producing ATP via anaerobic glycolysis, energy is in extremely limited supply and must be used as efficiently as possible (Kenney, Wilmore, and Costill 2022). High-intensity exercise for more than 40 minutes can deplete the glucose circulating in the blood as well as the glycogen stored in muscle cells. Once exercise is over, the involved muscles will have to replace the glycogen used to fuel activity so they can function at their optimal level of performance after an appropriate amount of recovery. Understanding when to consume carbohydrates at the completion of high-intensity exercise could help to quickly replace energy stores and speed up the recovery process.

Measuring the Intensity
of Metabolic Conditioning

Traditionally, measuring the intensity of metabolic conditioning workouts has been a function of identifying your target heart rate as a percentage of your age-predicted maximum heart rate (MHR, defined as 220 minus your age in years). For example, a 30-year-old would have an MHR of 190 beats per minute (220 − 30); exercising at 80 percent of that MHR would require maintaining a heart rate of 152 beats per minute (190 × 0.8). A review of the research related to heart-rate formulas, however, did not identify any specific source to validate this formula; many of the existing equations contain margins of error considered "unacceptably large" (Robergs and Landwehr 2002). A heart-rate monitor can help you train at a specific level of exercise intensity; however, using the formula of 220 minus your age, or similar formulas, only provides a guide for intensity and is not 100 percent relevant to your personal level of fitness. Nonetheless, identifying your heart rate at specific levels of intensity can help you to dial in your training on the precise metabolic energy pathway you want to develop.

The Talk Test

Rather than use an outdated, arbitrary formula to guess exercise intensity, the American Council on Exercise recommends using the talk test to estimate your exercise heart rate at a specific metabolic marker, which can help identify whether you are using fat or carbohydrates for fuel (Bryant, Merrill, and Green 2014). The talk test can estimate your heart rate at the point where working muscles transition from using aerobic to anaerobic metabolism for ATP production, a marker referred to as the first ventilatory threshold (VT_1). Identifying your heart rate at the VT_1 is relatively easy and can be done with the talk test while using a heart-rate monitor and treadmill; it can help you determine when you are using long-term energy pathways to metabolize fat or glycogen with oxygen or when your working muscles transition to anaerobic metabolism (using ATP stored in muscle cells or metabolizing glycogen to ATP without oxygen). Exercising at an intensity below the VT_1 helps to improve your aerobic efficiency, while exercising at an intensity above VT_1 could help to improve your ability to efficiently convert carbohydrates to ATP.

When you can talk comfortably, like when taking a walk or while during the warm-up phase of a workout, you are working at an intensity below the VT_1, and your working muscles are using the long-term energy pathways to metabolize oxygen and fat into ATP. When the intensity of exercise increases, muscle cells need energy immediately, causing the working muscles to begin producing ATP from glucose without oxygen (anaerobic metabolism). One result of the shift to anaerobic metabolism is the need to remove carbon dioxide (CO_2) faster from the lungs during the expiration (exhalation) phase of breathing, which explains why you breathe faster as you exercise harder—your lungs are trying to push out CO_2 while simultaneously trying to pull oxygen in. Think of CO_2 as the exhaust product of your muscles' use of glycogen for ATP; the faster you can push it out, the harder you might be able to work.

How to Conduct the Talk Test

As the intensity of exercise increases, ventilation (the rate at which we breathe) increases as well. As muscle cells transition from lipolysis to glycolysis to produce the ATP to fuel activity, your breathing rate will increase so that you can push more CO_2 out of your body and bring more oxygen in, which limits your ability to talk. Identifying your heart rate at this point, the VT_1, can help you to use a specific metabolic pathway when you exercise; exercising below the VT_1 uses aerobic respiration, and exercising above it relies on glycolysis or stored ATP. A talk test is a simple process. It requires a piece of exercise equipment like a treadmill, stationary bike, or elliptical runner that allows you to gradually and consistently increase the level of difficulty, along with a stopwatch, a heart-rate monitor, and a relatively brief passage you can say out loud, such as the U.S. Pledge of Allegiance or the "Happy Birthday" song.

The five steps of the talk test are below. For the most accurate results, it is best to conduct this test with a friend who can help monitor your heart rate as you progress from one stage to the next.

1. Begin with a three- to five-minute warm-up at a heart rate of less than 120 beats per minute or a rating of 3 or 4 out of 10 on the RPE scale. As you go through the following steps, it is essential that each stage of increasing exercise intensity should be the same duration.

2. At the completion of the warm-up, begin the first stage of exercise, which should be 60 to 120 seconds long.

3. During the last 30 seconds of the stage, sing the song "Happy Birthday" or say the Pledge of Allegiance out loud. Have your friend record your heart rate. (Note: If you are working aerobically, you should be able to easily complete either the song or the pledge. If breathing fast makes that challenging, you have crossed over the VT_1.)

4. After completing the phase, increase the level of difficulty. This could mean adding speed or incline on a treadmill or increasing the level of intensity on a stationary bike or elliptical runner; again, to be as accurate as possible, increase the intensity by the same amount each time. For example, if using incline on a treadmill, increase by a one-percent grade for each stage of the test.

5. Begin the next stage; during the last 30 seconds, repeat the song or the pledge while your friend records your heart rate. Upon completion of the song or pledge, increase the level of difficulty and begin the next stage. Repeat this process until speech becomes challenging and you can no longer say or sing the passage consistently from start to finish without pausing to catch your breath. This is an indication of VT_1; have your friend record that heart rate.

You now know your VT_1 heart rate. If you exercise at a lower intensity, aerobic respiration should provide the majority of the ATP required. If you exercise above that heart rate, your muscles will most likely be producing ATP through glycolysis.

Adapted from Bryant, Merrill, and Green (2014).

Onset of Blood Lactate

The second ventilatory threshold (VT_2), also known as the onset of blood lactate (OBLA) or lactate threshold, is the point where lactate, a by-product of anaerobic metabolism, starts accumulating in muscle cells. Exercising at the VT_2 can cause discomfort because lactate, along with other metabolites, can accumulate rapidly, causing the blood to become more acidic. Identifying your heart rate at the VT_2 requires a more specific test and is not necessarily required to perform high-intensity workouts. Breathing hard, barely being able to say one or two words at a time, and feeling a burning sensation in your muscles are indicators that you are working at an intensity near the VT_2. It is an intensity that allows you to sustain activity for only a brief period before needing a recovery interval to remove metabolic by-products and metabolize new ATP.

Think of your heart rate at the VT_2 or OBLA as similar to the redline on your car's tachometer (which measures the revolutions per minute while your engine is running); when you need to go fast to merge onto a highway, you can push your car to the redline for a brief amount of time, but keeping it there for too long could cause serious engine damage. This provides a rough but accurate analogy about exercise at the VT_2 or OBLA; it can be effective for a burst of speed, pushing to climb a hill, burning a lot of calories, or improving your ability to tolerate discomfort and exercise at the lactate threshold, but too much could result in overtraining, making it important to know how to measure intensity for metabolic conditioning.

Using the markers for the VT_1 and VT_2 gives you the information you need for designing metabolic conditioning workouts that could improve your ability to exercise using anaerobic metabolism (working near the VT_2) or enhance your ability to use oxygen to metabolize ATP (exercising at or near the VT_1). Tracking the intensity of your workouts allows you to design a program where a hard workout at the VT_2 could be followed by a lower-intensity workout at the VT_1 to help promote overall recovery.

Using a Wearable Device

When you have specific fitness or performance goals, a fitness tracker or heart-rate monitor becomes an essential piece of exercise equipment because it allows you to measure exactly how hard you are exercising. Having a heart-rate monitor can allow you to do the talk test and identify your heart rate at the VT_1. It also allows you to identify your heart rate at an estimate of your VT_2 (when you can feel your muscles really burning), which provides the information for designing a three-zone system of interval training for your metabolic conditioning workouts. Perform your hardest intervals at a heart rate above the VT_2, your moderate-intensity intervals at a heart rate above the VT_1 but below the VT_2, and your low-intensity intervals below the VT_1. This three-zone model can help you monitor your exercise intensity to get the results you want. Knowing exactly how hard you are working when you exercise will help you identify the most effective recovery strategies for your needs. In some cases, you will want to train at a high intensity, near the VT_2, to elevate your anaerobic threshold, while in other cases, you will want to train below the VT_1 to improve overall aerobic efficiency (the ability to deliver oxygen to working muscles). Using a wearable device gives you valuable insight into the overall efficiency of your training program.

Identifying the Best Wearable Device for Your Needs

Heart-rate monitors have been used for years to measure and record heart-rate data during exercise. However, it's only been in the past decade or so that watches used as heart-rate monitors have become a part of our daily wardrobe. Fitness trackers, smartwatches, monitors, rings, arm bands—there are a variety of different wearable devices, which can make it a challenge to identify the best one for your needs. Here are a few questions to consider:

- *What are you training for and what data do you want to record?* The activity you're training for will dictate the data you want to record. For example, if you're training for a powerlifting meet, you're probably more interested in learning about sleep and recovery than monitoring your heart rate during training, whereas if you're training for a marathon, you might want to record your heart rate during your workouts while also being able to track data while you sleep to ensure optimal recovery.

- *Do you want to be able to monitor and track your sleep?* Sleep is when your muscles are actually going through the repair process. A tracker that can monitor sleep could help you to dial in an important component of the recovery process so that you get the optimal sleep for your needs.

- *Do you like being motivated by friends or training partners?* If seeing what your friends are doing for their workouts is important for your motivation, consider using a tracker that links to an app where you can connect with friends. This way, when your friends record and post a training session, it's a reminder for your own workout.

- *What type of device do you want to wear?* From arm bands, watches, and chest straps to rings and specially designed shirts, there are a number of devices that can record your heart rate, both while you're training and during your normal daily activities. You have to decide which you prefer wearing and which records the data most relevant to your needs.

- *Do you like the app interface?* Are the recorded data easy to access and understand? Can you easily use the interface to identify trends, bad or good, that could influence the outcome of your training program? No matter which wearable device you select, it will have a companion smartphone app, and you want to make sure that app is easy to navigate and records the information most relevant to your needs.

- *What is the battery life?* Read the manufacturer's listing *and* product reviews; a wearable device could look great and provide good data, but a limited battery life could hamper its ultimate usability.

As you shop for a wearable device, read the reviews of previous buyers, both good and bad, to get a sense of whether it can be an effective resource for your training needs. No matter which device you buy, it's only effective if you use the data you record. That's where the app comes in—it should allow you to review training logs and calendars to identify trends so you can adjust your program accordingly.

Regardless of whether a resistance training program uses 85 percent of the 1RM or 10RM or a metabolic conditioning program uses a specific percentage of the maximum heart rate, the markers for the VT_1 and VT_2, or the RPE, it is important to have a system that allows you to monitor how hard you are working when you exercise. For best results, it is not necessary to work at the highest level of intensity all the time; lower-intensity workouts can help improve aerobic efficiency as well as be effective for active recovery that can promote the repair process the day after a grueling workout. Table 2.1 identifies markers for the varying levels of intensity you could experience during a workout, along with an estimate of the recovery time for training at that intensity.

TABLE 2.1 Measuring the Intensity of Exercise

LEVEL OF INTENSITY	RATING OF PERCEIVED EXERTION, ON A SCALE OF 1-10	METABOLIC MARKERS AND PATHWAYS	ESTIMATED PERCENTAGE OF MAXIMUM HEART RATE	STRENGTH TRAINING REPETITION MAXIMUM (RM)[a]	ESTIMATED DURATION OF RECOVERY[b]
Very low	1-4	Below VT_1 (aerobic respiration)	50-59	20RM	None
Low	5-6	At VT_1 (aerobic glycolysis)	60-69	12RM-20RM	Less than 24 hours
Moderate	7-8	Above VT_1 and below VT_2 (aerobic and anaerobic glycolysis)	70-84	6RM-12RM	24-48 hours
High	9-10	VT_2 or above (anaerobic ATP-PC)	85-100	1RM-6RM	48-72 hours

Abbreviations: ATP, adenosine triphosphate; PC, phosphocreatine; VT_1, first ventilatory threshold; VT_2, second ventilatory threshold.

[a]Repetition maximum means the number of repetitions performed to reach a point of fatigue; for example, 10RM indicates an intensity that causes fatigue at 10 repetitions.

[b]The type of exercise performed, along with the level of intensity and amount of muscle mass activated during the workout, will influence the length of the recovery process.

How Moderate- to High-Intensity Exercise Affects Your Body

At this point, you're aware of the benefits of high-intensity exercise but may not be familiar with how it affects your muscles and the ability to recover before your next hard workout. The stark reality is that what you do after a high-intensity workout is over can be the difference between getting results or simply spinning your wheels with nothing to show for it. It could take anywhere from

24 to 72 hours to fully recover from an extremely demanding workout, and the types of muscle contractions performed can influence the amount and type of soreness the day after. One reason is because high-intensity exercise changes the biochemistry of your muscle tissue, which could result in overall fatigue if not properly addressed. For example, calcium is an electrolyte that facilitates the electrical charge responsible for signaling muscle motor units to contract. Calcium pumping, the process of delivering calcium to the cells to facilitate the signal for contraction, is estimated to account for up to 80 percent of the energy cost of a muscle contraction (Cheng, Jude, and Lanner 2020). A loss of calcium could contribute to the sense of overall fatigue and keep a muscle from being able to achieve an optimal level of performance.

In addition, high-intensity exercise results in muscle damage because it relies on anaerobic metabolism, specifically either stored ATP or ATP metabolized from glucose without the presence of oxygen. These sources of ATP result in a number of by-products referred to as metabolites, including hydrogen ions, inorganic phosphates, and lactic acid, which can accumulate in muscle tissue and interfere with a muscle's ability to produce force. For example, the explosive contractions required for sports that require rapid starts, stops, and changes of direction create a different amount of damage than the steady, consistent contractions of a lower-intensity, endurance-oriented activity. Too many challenging workouts scheduled too close together may not allow time for your body to rest, replace lost energy stores, or rebuild new muscle tissue.

The Role of Inflammation Immediately After Exercise

Acute inflammation localized in the involved muscle tissues is a normal response to high-intensity exercise and is the result of the immune system releasing leukocytes (white blood cells) to clean up and eliminate the metabolites created by high-intensity exercise. In general, when a disease, infection, or outside invader is introduced to the body, the initial response is to increase leukocyte levels to eliminate the threat. Inflammation occurs as the result of leukocytes, macrophages, and other immune cells that help repair tissues and remove waste products or damaged cells. Leukocyte levels have been observed to remain elevated for the first 3 hours after exercise; at 12 hours, they can be up to 30 percent higher than normal resting levels, with a complete return to normal resting levels by 24 hours after the workout. Levels of macrophages and neutrophils, which remove damaged cells, can remain elevated for up to 24 hours after exercise (Bessa et al. 2016). Acute inflammation can interfere with a muscle's ability to contract and could last up to 24 hours; therefore, when playing multievent tournaments, it is important to manage inflammation as well as possible so that the muscles can achieve their optimal level of performance.

Biomarkers of Muscle Damage

The amount and severity of muscle damage will influence the levels of metabolites and biomarkers produced. Elevated levels of these biomarkers and metabolites can impede energy metabolism and interfere with a muscle's ability to contract, helping to explain those feelings of general fatigue and soreness in your muscles the day after a hard workout. During exercise, cell membranes become more permeable, which can allow enzymes such as creatine kinase (CK) or lactate dehydrogenase to leak into surrounding cell fluid, and ultimately, the circulatory

Rhabdomyolysis

In 2011, during a conditioning session, 13 members of the University of Iowa football team experienced rhabdomyolysis, a serious medical condition that occurs when muscle tissue is damaged and releases proteins and electrolytes into the bloodstream. After playing in a bowl game in late December 2010, the players had a three-week break from training. In late January 2011, at the first few conditioning sessions back from the break, they were required to perform sled pushes in addition to completing 100 back squats with 50 percent of their body weight and other weightlifting activities. As a result of the high volume of conditioning after a three-week break, 13 players were admitted to the hospital to be treated for rhabdomyolysis. Dr. Ned Amendola, MD, director of the University of Iowa Sports Medicine Center and team physician for the football team, was a coauthor of a study that reviewed the incident to identify how to best avoid any similar situations in the future. He said of the incident, "Coaches should be aware that, if athletes are coming back to camp or school and need to get back in shape, the training sessions should proceed gradually" (McKee 2013). A surprising finding of the review was the effect of protein supplementation. "Interestingly, we found that protein shakes consumed during the day of the workout or the day before the workout seem to protect the muscle from getting injured," Amendola said (McKee 2013).

Unfortunately, this is not the only situation where high-intensity training has put athletes at risk. Scenes like this happen in all levels of sport. If you're an athlete, the point is to recognize the difference between normal fatigue and the level of exertion that gets beyond uncomfortable. You no doubt thrive on discomfort, but it's important to know when the high-intensity line has been crossed for too long, because it could ultimately impede your overall training efforts. Another point is for coaches: When returning to conditioning after a few weeks off, it is best to start with a lower volume and intensity and gradually increase over a series of workouts, as opposed to programming the first workout of a break to pick up where you left off before it. No matter how well athletes followed the off-season conditioning program prepared for them, they will need a few workouts to transition back to the normal training intensity.

system. In addition, levels of biomarkers such as reactive oxygen species, CK, and myoglobin indicate muscle damage and can remain elevated for up to 36 hours after high-intensity exercise (Bessa et al. 2016; Cheng, Jude, and Lanner 2020). Excessive amounts of CK and myoglobin in the bloodstream could cause exertional rhabdomyolysis and result in kidney (renal) failure or even death (Cheng, Jude, and Lanner 2020).

Immediately after a high-intensity workout, your circulatory system is removing the by-products of anaerobic metabolism while delivering immune cells, glucose, oxygen, and other vital components necessary for repairing tissue and replacing energy. Besides resulting in lactic acid, high-intensity exercise elevates levels of hydrogen ions and other by-products of anaerobic metabolism; this increases blood acidity, referred to as acidosis, and reduces the levels of oxygen and other nutrients available for aerobic energy production. In extreme cases, acidosis can cause severe damage to muscle tissue, resulting in a breakdown of muscle protein called myoglobin. When myoglobin is broken down and subsequently enters the bloodstream, this could ultimately lead to rhabdomyolysis. Rhabdomyolysis can inhibit normal function of the kidneys, potentially leading to hospitalization or possibly death, so it is extremely important to listen to your body and not push physical exertion past your normal comfort levels.

Sodium is an essential electrolyte that helps increase the permeability of cell membranes to allow water and oxygen into the cell while metabolites and markers of muscle damage are removed. In a muscle cell, glycogen is attached to water. As glycogen is metabolized into ATP, the water is released to help control the body's internal temperature; this causes sweat, which contains sodium, to accumulate on the skin. Once the workout is over, hydration, especially hydration containing electrolytes to replace those such as sodium that are lost in sweat, can help restore intracellular water levels and promote the removal of damaging metabolites to minimize fatigue while your muscles return to optimal function.

Table 2.2 identifies how high-intensity exercise damages muscles and creates a sense of fatigue at the end of a hard workout.

The Effect of Intensity

Exercise is the application of physical stress, and that stress makes specific changes to the cells and structures of your tissues. This chapter addressed how high-intensity exercise affects your muscles from the cellular level up. If you use high-intensity exercise to reach your goals, avoid becoming overtrained by developing a system to monitor and record the intensity of your workouts so you know when to allow for appropriate rest. Different levels of intensity affect the tissues and structures of your body in different ways; monitoring your training intensity and understanding how this stress affects your ability to perform can help you identify the most appropriate recovery method to meet the needs of your specific workout program. Recording the intensity of your workouts, along with how you feel throughout the immediate postworkout recovery period, can help you develop the most effective recovery-based training program for your needs.

TABLE 2.2 Types of Metabolic Damage

METABOLIC DAMAGE	EFFECTS
Elevated blood lactate	When muscles involved in exercise can no longer meet energy demands through aerobic metabolism during moderate- to high-intensity exercise, muscle cells will metabolize ATP via anaerobic glycolysis. One by-product of anaerobic metabolism is lactate, which can accumulate quickly during high-intensity exercise. The OBLA is a marker indicating an elevation in blood acidity and is also referred to as the lactate threshold. Elevated levels of lactate can restrict the ability of muscle cells to produce ATP, one possible cause of the fatigue experienced during hard exercise. That burning sensation you feel in your muscles during high-intensity exercise is an indication of OBLA and a sign that it is time for a lower-intensity active recovery interval. However, regular HIIT can improve overall fitness by training muscles to tolerate working at the OBLA as well as enhancing the ability to quickly remove lactate and other metabolites that accumulate as the result of anaerobic metabolism.
Acidosis	Besides blood lactate, anaerobic metabolism also elevates levels of hydrogen ions, which can increase overall blood acidity. In extreme cases, acidosis can cause severe damage to muscle tissue, resulting in a breakdown of muscle protein called myoglobin. An accumulation of myoglobin in the bloodstream could ultimately result in rhabdomyolysis. Rhabdomyolysis can inhibit normal function of the kidneys, potentially leading to hospitalization (and in extreme cases, death), making it extremely important to listen to your body and not push physical exertion past your comfort level.
Gluconeogenesis	Exercise signals the production of cortisol, a steroid hormone produced by the adrenal glands in response to stress, low blood sugar, and exercise. Muscle cells normally use free fatty acids and glucose to produce ATP, saving protein to be used for repairing muscle and connective tissues damaged during exercise. Carbohydrates are stored as glycogen in muscle cells and the liver until they are needed for ATP production during strenuous exercise (glycogen must first be converted to glucose before it can be fully metabolized to ATP). At rest and during low-intensity exercise, muscle cells create ATP from aerobic respiration, the long-term energy pathway. However, aerobic respiration can take a relatively long time to produce ATP, making it an inefficient energy source during high-intensity exercise. Both aerobic and anaerobic glycolysis can produce ATP more quickly than aerobic respiration; however, during periods of extended moderate- to high-intensity exercise, muscle cells can deplete available carbohydrates. When glucose is not available for ATP, cortisol, normally used to metabolize fat and carbohydrates to ATP, can metabolize protein into glucose (for ATP) via a process called gluconeogenesis. This, in turn, can reduce the amount of protein available for tissue repair. In addition, elevated levels of cortisol could inhibit protein synthesis, reduce the inflammation essential for postexercise tissue repair, and elevate levels of ammonia in the blood, increasing blood acidity while reducing the ability of muscles to function efficiently (Kenney, Wilmore, and Costill 2022).

Abbreviations: ATP, adenosine triphosphate; HIIT, high-intensity interval training; OBLA, onset of blood lactate.

3

SYSTEMS OVERLOAD

You don't need to be an automotive engineer to know that all the systems in your car—the starter motor, the engine, the drivetrain, the steering, and of course, the brakes—have to perform at an optimal level of function to ensure your safety. In addition, you probably recognize that a lot of strenuous, stop-and-go city driving will place more stress on these systems than cruising on a rural highway at a steady pace. In many ways, exercise is the same; a lot of high-intensity exercise will place a lot of wear and tear on various systems in your body, like the muscular, metabolic, and endocrine systems. When you use your car for city driving, you know you should budget more money for repairs and maintenance so that it performs to the best of its ability. The same is true for high-intensity exercise; when you plan a phase of high-intensity exercise, you should also plan the appropriate recovery strategies in an effort to achieve optimal adaptation. By reading this book, you are developing the knowledge of how high-intensity exercise places a lot of stress on the various systems of the body, and you are beginning to understand the role that rest, along with lower-intensity exercise, should play in your overall workout program.

Homeostasis

As you read these words, you're probably sitting in a quiet place and have opened this book with the expectation of learning a little bit more about how your body responds to exercise. Right now, at this moment, your heart is working to pump oxygenated blood around your body and to move deoxygenated blood back to your lungs so the carbon dioxide can be removed and new oxygen can be placed in the bloodstream. Because you are not physically moving while reading these words, you are not exerting much energy; your muscle cells only need to metabolize a minimal amount of energy to function properly. This is the state of relative rest known as homeostasis, the technical term for the normal operating condition of the human body. When your body is in homeostasis, your muscles are consuming approximately 3.5 milliliters of oxygen per kilogram of your body weight (0.05 fl oz/lb); as soon as you start moving, whether to go for a run, perform some household chores, or play power forward for the Lakers, your muscles will need oxygen and energy so they have the ability to produce force for the intended activity, and your body will no longer be in homeostasis.

Exercise Is Stress

Stress, whether emotional or physical, disrupts homeostasis and initiates a number of physiological reactions, such as the release of various hormones, that allow your body to produce the energy required to respond to the stress stimulus. Strenuous physical activity such as moderate- to high-intensity exercise is a specific type of stress that disrupts homeostasis by requiring muscle cells to metabolize the energy to fuel force production. When muscle cells produce energy to fuel the contractions required to move the body, heat is generated and internal temperatures are elevated. Once exercise is over, the body will go through the process of returning to homeostasis, and this is a time when circulation, responsible for pumping oxygen-carrying blood to working muscles during exercise, is returning to normal. Depending on the intensity and duration of the workout, the body's internal temperature slowly returns to normal, while circulation remains elevated above resting levels in order to move oxygenated and nutrient-carrying blood to the muscles involved in exercise as they replace energy and restore hydration in muscle cells.

The EPOC Effect

Even though the workout might be over, after strenuous exercise, your muscles continue expending energy to replace energy (specifically, the glycogen and adenosine triphosphate [ATP] used during exercise for anaerobic metabolism), to repair damaged tissues, and to remove metabolic by-products, all of which can be identified by elevated levels of oxygen consumption, technically referred to as excess postexercise oxygen consumption (EPOC).

Here's a cool fact: The human body burns approximately five calories of energy to consume one liter (1 qt) of oxygen; the more muscles involved in exercise, the greater the oxygen consumption and subsequent caloric expenditure (Kenney, Wilmore, and Costill 2022).

This explains how your body continues to burn calories after a workout is over, because during EPOC, the involved muscles are consuming a higher volume of oxygen while returning to homeostasis. In a review of the research, Dupuy and colleagues (2018, 2) describe the recovery process as a "return to homeostasis of physiological systems following metabolic and muscle damage induced by exercise." The purpose of applying a specific recovery strategy is to promote the return to homeostasis, which in turn facilitates your body's ability to prepare for the next workout or competition.

Stress and the Nervous System

High-intensity exercise results in two types of overload on the muscle and connective tissues of the myofascial system: metabolic and mechanical.

1. *Metabolic overload.* Metabolic overload is the process of depleting muscle cells of available energy. Type II muscle fibers store glycogen and ATP to fuel contractions; high-intensity exercise depletes these resources, and it takes

time to replace them so muscles are properly fueled for the next workout (or competition). The volume and intensity of exercise to create metabolic overload often results in an accumulation of by-products, including inorganic phosphates, hydrogen ions, and lactate. As these accumulate in the blood of working muscles, it can lead to feelings of soreness and fatigue.

2. *Mechanical overload.* Mechanical overload creates physical damage to the protein structures of individual muscle fibers and connective tissues. As a result of this damage, fibroblasts produced in the sarcolemma of muscle cells are used to repair the structures damaged by physical exertion.

Exercise at an intensity high enough to create mechanical or metabolic overload can also affect the function of the nervous system. The central nervous system includes the brain and spinal cord and more than 100 billion neurons, all of which are influenced by stress, such as excessive amounts of exercise. The peripheral nervous system, a main component of the central nervous system, contains both sensory and motor neurons; the sensory neurons identify both

The Role of Hormones in the Recovery Process

Hormones are chemicals released by glands and organs that control how cells (and in turn, all of the tissues in the body) function. Some hormones, such as cortisol, are involved in producing the energy for exercise, whereas other hormones play essential roles in the process of postexercise recovery. The initial adaptations from a strength training program are neural, meaning that muscle motor units are becoming more effective at stimulating muscle fibers to contract. However, over the long term of an exercise program, the hormones produced by the endocrine system are what can have the greatest influence on how your body adapts. Hormones can be either anabolic, meaning they promote tissue growth, or catabolic, meaning they function to break down nutrients, cells, or other structures in the body. Chapter 9 will have more information on the hormones related to energy metabolism; meanwhile, high-intensity exercise that causes mechanical damage to tissues or metabolic stress to muscle cells stimulates the production of anabolic hormones responsible for repairing the proteins that compose muscle, fascia, and elastic connective tissues. Among other functions, human growth hormone (HGH), insulin-like growth factor 1 (IGF-1), and testosterone help repair damaged muscle proteins and play an essential role in increasing muscle size and enhancing force output.

Hormones have both short- and long-term responses to high-intensity exercise that can help determine how quickly your muscles recover. In the acute phase immediately after exercise, testosterone, HGH, and IGF-1 are released to repair the proteins of damaged muscle and connective tissues. During a long-term exercise program, there will be an increase in both the levels of circulating hormones and the receptor sites in muscle cells that allow testosterone, HGH, and IGF-1 to perform their functions. Exercise performed to a point of momentary fatigue will generate high levels of both the mechanical and the metabolic stress that damage muscle proteins and signal the release of testosterone, HGH, and IGF-1 to repair the damaged tissues.

internal and external stimuli to determine an appropriate response by motor neurons and the muscle fibers they activate. High-intensity exercise can fatigue the peripheral nervous system and could result in faulty motor output, which could subsequently cause an injury.

The autonomic nervous system is considered a component of the peripheral nervous system's motor system and regulates involuntary functions including heart rate, lung function, blood circulation, and blood pressure. The autonomic nervous system contains two components: the sympathetic nervous system (SNS) and the parasympathetic nervous system (PNS), each of which have a direct effect on the return to homeostasis after exercise.

Sympathetic Nervous System

The SNS is activated in response to stress; it releases hormones and neurotransmitters, including cortisol, epinephrine, and norepinephrine, which help to elevate the heart rate, regulate energy production, dilate blood vessels for easier blood transport to working muscles, and boost cardiac output. The SNS is often called the fight-or-flight system because it engages at the first sign of any immediate stress, whether that is lifting a heavy barbell, driving the lane during a basketball game, or keeping your child from running into the street. An accumulation of physical fatigue, combined with the activation of the SNS, could influence your body's ability to recover from high-intensity exercise.

Increased SNS activity during rest, which could cause an elevated heart rate or disrupt your ability to fall asleep even though you feel exhausted, is an indication of sympathetic overtraining, thought to be caused by increased neural activity resulting from the magnitude of motor unit recruitment required to generate high levels of force from high-intensity strength or power exercises (Haff and Triplett 2016). When you are lying in bed, completely exhausted, yet your heart is racing and you can't get to sleep, that is an indication of an overactive SNS; too many high-intensity strength, power, or metabolic conditioning workouts combined with inadequate rest, refueling, and rehydration in between each session could result in sympathetic overtraining (Kenney, Wilmore, and Costill 2022).

Signs of Sympathetic Overtraining

Increased resting heart rate

Increased blood pressure

Loss of appetite

Loss of body mass

Sleep disturbances

Change in emotional and mood state

Parasympathetic Nervous System

The PNS works opposite of the SNS and has earned the nickname "the rest and digest system." The PNS controls involuntary functions such as glandular secretion (important for the hormones that help repair damaged muscles), urination (important for removing the by-products from anaerobic metabolism), regulation of the heart rate, and constriction of blood vessels, all of which help the body to return to homeostasis.

Excessive training could result in parasympathetic overtraining, which suppresses normal function of many of the body's physiological systems. If you perform an excessive volume of low- to moderate-intensity endurance training without adequate rest, refueling, or rehydration, you could be at risk of developing parasympathetic overtraining (Kenney, Wilmore, and Costill 2022).

Signs of Parasympathetic Overtraining

Early onset of fatigue

Low resting heart rate

Rapid heart-rate recovery after exercise

Low resting blood pressure

Underrecovered, Not Overtrained

Recall the symptoms and effects of overtraining syndrome (OTS), discussed in detail in chapter 1. There is a limit to the amount of physical overload the systems of the body can experience before becoming overworked, and an accumulation of exercise fatigue could ultimately result in OTS along with a number of undesired physical changes, including weight gain, a loss of muscle mass, or a weakened immune system, each of which could derail your fitness efforts and keep you from reaching your goals (Bishop, Jones, and Woods 2008; Hausswirth and Mujika 2013; Wyatt, Donaldson, and Brown 2013). The volume or mode of exercise alone is not the cause of OTS; rather, it is a combination of a lack of proper rest, inadequate nutrition to refuel after exercise, and poor hydration between high-intensity workouts. Thus, when you are feeling tired and fatigued, identify it as being underrecovered as opposed to overtrained. To create the optimal adaptations from your workouts, when you plan high-intensity exercise or design a program that will emphasize a high volume of exercise in a relatively short period of time, also plan appropriate strategies to promote optimal postworkout recovery.

Different Types of Overload

Exercise is when the body experiences mechanical and metabolic overload. Exercise for the purpose of elevating the heart rate while challenging muscle cells to metabolize the energy required for contractions is a metabolic stress that affects primarily your cardiorespiratory and muscular systems. High-intensity exercise, such as heavy strength training or explosive power training, applies tremendous amounts of mechanical stress to tissues and skeletal structures. Exercise to the point of fatigue is the process of applying both types of stress, and the recovery period *after* exercise is when your body repairs damaged tissues, replaces ATP used by muscle cells to fuel muscle-force production, and otherwise allows all of its systems to return to homeostasis.

Every workout or competition initiates a number of short-term responses in your body; when exercise is performed consistently, these responses ultimately result in long-term changes. The short-term responses take place either during or immediately after a workout and gradually accumulate into long-term changes to your body. One example of an immediate response to a workout is localized muscle fatigue resulting from applying mechanical forces and depleting the ATP stored in muscle cells. Long-term adaptations only occur after consistent exposure to a specific type of exercise during the course of a program. As one example of a long-term adaptation, muscle cells adapt to store more glycogen (and water) to provide more energy during exercise while at the same time improving the ability to produce sodium bicarbonate to reduce blood acidity, both of which help to delay the point of fatigue during high-intensity exercise.

Sufficient rest is required between challenging workouts, because your muscles need time to rehydrate, refuel, and rest so they have the ability to function at a high level of performance the next time they are called into action. For your body to achieve an optimal level of performance during the course of a week, you probably want to have two to three high-intensity workouts, two to three moderate-intensity workouts, and one to three low-intensity workouts. No, you can't add days to the calendar to make a nine-day week; there will be some weeks when you're achieving an optimal amount of rest and nutrition and you can knock out three challenging workouts, whereas during other weeks, life might get in the way and keep you from getting the sleep you need or interrupt your ability to consume healthy nutrition, and you may only be able to handle one really hard workout and a couple of moderate-intensity ones. During a stressful period at home or work, it's best to take a break from high-intensity exercise, because it could result in too much stress being applied to your body. When life becomes stressful and overwhelming, sometimes the best exercise you can do is to just get outside for a long walk or do a low-intensity bodyweight workout for mobility, both of which help to elevate circulation to promote recovery and reduce overall levels of stress.

Overload and Pain

Pain is a sharp, extremely uncomfortable sensation signaling that the body is experiencing too much physical stress, and whatever activity you're doing should be stopped immediately. Discomfort, on the other hand, is the goal of moderate- to high-intensity exercise and is merely an indication that muscles have worked beyond their existing ability. Discomfort means your body is being challenged to work harder than it is used to working, whereas pain is an indication that your body is experiencing an acute overload of stress that could cause an injury; when it comes to exercise, you want the former but definitely not the latter. However, exercise to the point of discomfort is a signal that muscles will need time to repair and refuel before they can be challenged again.

Balance Between Stress and Rest

One way to think about performing high-intensity exercise is that you're trying to become comfortable with being physically uncomfortable, because being able to tolerate that discomfort could give you an edge over your competition or help you meet your fitness goals. However, when you do the tough workouts that cause discomfort, you will also want to apply the recovery strategies that can alleviate it as soon as possible. Discomfort is a signal that your body is being pushed to new boundaries that should cause the physical changes you want from a workout program, but it's also a signal that your body will need to recharge before the next bout of strenuous activity.

Case Study: Overcoming Overtraining

Amanda is a personal trainer and competitive triathlete. In the mid-2010s, she experienced a thyroid nodule that grew to three times its original size and restricted oxygen intake into her body. "I believe that high-intensity exercise combined with inadequate sleep and teaching as many fitness classes as I could in a single week while only fueling with granola bars and protein shakes was not sustainable and could have killed me if I kept following that path," she said. According to Amanda, she was constantly tired before her diagnosis, but the more tired she was, the harder she pushed herself to train, resulting in a complete overload on her endocrine system.

After her health scare, Amanda committed to training smarter, not harder. As she prepared for her most recent attempt at the Kona Ironman, she followed a very structured training schedule that progressed from 12 to 25 hours a week during the buildup to the race. Now, as a result of her experience, Amanda will take one day a week off when preparing for a race; the only activity is an easy run or bike ride at a very low intensity, just enough to make her breathe a little harder. She follows a schedule of three build weeks followed by a recovery week of lower-intensity exercise, with most of her training at moderate intensity so she can focus on aerobic energy production. Amanda tracks her training volume using a training stress score that rates the intensity of each training session; this helps her to monitor her intensity and allow for adequate rest between hard training days. Her favorite recovery strategy is monitoring her resting heart rate and heart-rate variability; any deviation from normal is an indication to adjust training, rest, or both. In addition, Amanda emphasizes her sleep hygiene while preparing for a race; she knows how good she feels after a long sleep and uses that to ensure optimal recovery between hard training days. Amanda is grateful for her health scare, because it helped her to recognize that she was overtraining and needed to focus on recovery as part of her overall training regimen.

All Stress Accumulates

You may not be a professional athlete playing 162 baseball games, 82 basketball games, or 17 football games in a season, but you no doubt have many stressors in your life, and exercise is just another one. Feeling stressed or burned out, not being able to complete a workout due to fatigue, or having a tough time falling asleep even though you are physically exhausted are all signs of overtraining and a definite indicator that you need to apply specific recovery strategies after your workouts. The following chapters will provide strategies that can be applied immediately after workouts, the day after a hard training session, and long term, in addition to identifying a number of healthy habits that can promote optimal postworkout recovery when practiced consistently. Whatever your reason for training, it is important to understand that while you may *want* to push through a tough workout when you're feeling exhausted, sometimes the best thing you can do is to skip the hard workout and replace it with an easy, low-intensity one or take a complete rest day, because when it comes to exercise, there are times when less is more. Yes, high-intensity workouts can cause desired changes, but probably the most important day in your training schedule is the one most often overlooked—the rest day. Rest is necessary to allow your muscles to fully recover from the stresses of hard exercise, providing essential time for repair and growth.

Exercise should challenge you to work harder than your current abilities, but not every workout has to make you sore to be effective. As discussed in chapters 1 and 2, high-intensity exercise results in metabolic by-products, which can contribute to the sensation of discomfort characteristic of delayed-onset muscle soreness. When your muscles are feeling really sore, it is necessary to allow your circulatory system to perform its job of removing the metabolic by-products in muscle cells while delivering the oxygen and nutrients used to help repair damaged tissues, which can explain the benefits of low-intensity activity during the postexercise recovery process. Low-intensity exercise can elevate circulation so that tissues damaged from the mechanical stresses of exercise can be repaired and energy stores replaced in muscle cells. An easy workout is not a sign of being lazy; instead, exercising at a lower intensity provides your muscles with a chance to repair and refuel so you can be completely recovered before your next challenging workout or competition.

Exercise and the Immune System

Inadequate recovery can weaken the body's immune system. Illness is the second leading cause of missing practice or playing time for athletes, which has led to a field of study known as exercise immunology; as a result, researchers have developed a good understanding about how exercise can enhance or suppress the immune system (Peake et al. 2017; Simpson et al. 2015).

Scientists have identified a J-shaped curve that explains how exercise stress can accumulate to affect the immune system. A reasonable amount of moderate-intensity exercise could provide benefits for strengthening the immune system; however, too much exercise at too high of an intensity, combined with inadequate recovery time, could weaken the immune system, making the body more susceptible to infection (Gleeson 2007; Halabchi, Ahmadinejad, and Selk-Ghaffari 2020). As Gleeson (2007) notes, "While engaging in moderate activity may enhance immune function above sedentary levels, excessive amounts of prolonged, high-intensity exercise may impair immune function" (693).

The purpose of the immune system is to protect the body from foreign invaders that could cause a disease or otherwise disrupt homeostasis. Lymphocytes and macrophages are examples of cells produced by the body to neutralize and eliminate any outside bacteria or germs that could cause disease. Inflammation is a normal physiological response that indicates the immune system is functioning to eliminate a disruption to homeostasis. During exercise, the SNS and hypothalamus-pituitary-adrenal axis support energy metabolism; however, they also have an important effect on the immune system's ability to release the leukocytes and other cells responsible for fighting infections. Acute or short-term inflammation is part of the normal postexercise recovery process; after a single bout of moderate-intensity exercise, levels of leukocytes can increase, helping to strengthen the immune system (Simpson et al. 2015).

How many times have you had a lingering cold that wouldn't go away or an injury that wouldn't seem to heal? Continuing to participate in high-intensity exercise while sick or injured could overload your immune system and render it ineffective, and the only solution for getting better is rest. Simpson and colleagues (2020) wrote, "The impact of exercise on innate and acquired immune parameters is dependent on the intensity of exercise, the duration and overall load of training" (9). The effect of exercise on the immune system is based on multiple factors that help to regulate immune system function, including genetics, age, nutrition, training status, underlying health conditions, psychological stress, and medical history (Peake et al. 2017; Simpson et al. 2020).

Inflammation's Role in Exercise Recovery

During high-intensity muscle contractions, membranes of muscle cells become more permeable to allow for the transfer of fluid in and out of the cell. This increased permeability can allow metabolites and other by-products of anaerobic metabolism into the bloodstream. Another outcome of high-intensity muscle contractions is damage to structures called Z-lines, which connect series of individual sarcomeres, the smallest units of a muscle fiber. The components of a muscle fiber are arranged in series and attached via Z-lines; high-intensity contractions can damage the Z-lines between series of sarcomeres, and this damage initiates the body's automatic repair response—inflammation. Inflammation is an indication that the immune system is functioning properly; in the case of damaged muscle fibers, immune cells called macrophages and neutrophils will repair or remove damaged cells (Cheng, Jude, and Lanner 2020; Lee et al. 2017).

Inflammation *Is* Recovery

The postexercise soreness you feel and the inflammation you experience are indicators that your immune system is undergoing the normal repair process. The inflammation can trigger nociceptors, sensory receptors for pain, and make movement uncomfortable; specific strategies such as cryotherapy or sitting in an infrared sauna could help reduce inflammation and mitigate any perceived soreness. This acute inflammation is part of the normal repair process and an indication that your immune system is functioning properly. More importantly, this response from the immune system explains why it is so critical to allow an appropriate amount of time, approximately 48 to 72 hours, between high-intensity workouts involving the same muscles or movement patterns; your physiology, specifically your immune system, requires time to allow the healing process to occur. Performing moderate- to high-intensity exercise again before letting the body completely return to homeostasis could increase the risk of developing a virus or infection and, ultimately, overtraining syndrome (Peake et al. 2017).

Like many things in the human body, a little inflammation is good for you. It is a sign that your immune system is functioning to restore homeostasis. Chronic, or long-term, inflammation is a different story. Chronic inflammation could overwhelm your immune system and leave it susceptible to a virus or infection. One important benefit of an appropriate amount of time between high-intensity workouts is ensuring that your immune system is strong enough to support the recovery process *and* maintain the ability to fight any outside germ that tries to attack your body. As Cheng, Jude, and Lanner (2020) observed, "Repeated strenuous physical activity with too short recovery periods that [induce] soluble factors that [prolong] duration of inflammation will most certainly lead to decreased muscle function and may well be a key component in OTS" (6).

Recovery Timing and Immune Response

When it comes to extensive periods of high-intensity exercise or competitions, researchers have identified what they term an open window—when the immune system is compromised, increasing the likelihood of an infection entering the body (Peake et al. 2017; Simpson et al. 2015). According to Gleeson (2007), "Various immune cell functions are temporarily impaired following acute bouts of prolonged, continuous heavy exercise, and athletes engaged in intensive periods of endurance training appear to be more susceptible to minor infections" (693). Peake and colleagues (2017) noted, "If exercise is repeated again while the immune system is still depressed, this could lead to a greater degree of immunodepression and potentially a longer window of opportunity for infection" (1077). Simpson and colleagues (2020) observed that "arduous bouts of exercise, typically those practiced by athletes and other high-performance personnel (e.g. the military), have been associated with suppressed mucosal and cellular immunity, increased symptoms of upper respiratory tract infections (URTI), latent viral reactivation, and impaired immune responses to vaccine and novel antigens" (9).

The good news is that the research literature is overwhelmingly conclusive: limited moderate-intensity exercise (less than 45 minutes per day) can enhance the immune system and reduce the risk of becoming sick (Gleeson 2007; Halabchi, Ahmadinejad, and Selk-Ghaffari 2020; Hoffman 2014; Peake et al. 2017; Simpson et al. 2020; Simpson et al. 2015). However, unless you are training for a specific competition, it is a good idea to adjust the duration and reduce the intensity of exercise when it is cold and during flu season to ensure that your immune system remains as strong as the rest of the body.

Nutrition's Role in the Immune Response

Proper nutrition is essential for promoting optimal immune system performance. For example, carbohydrates ingested during and immediately after exercise could help support optimal immune function (Peake et al. 2017). This section is a brief review of nutrition to make the point that it is not a good idea to reduce or limit carbohydrate intake when performing extensive periods of high-intensity physical activity. This section also touches on how nutrient timing can help you to properly fuel, both for your workouts and for postexercise recovery. Exercise can also affect the immune system by limiting the availability of glycogen for metabolism of immune cells. According to Simpson and colleagues (2020), "Immuno-metabolism is an emerging science that highlights connections between the metabolic state of immune cells and the nature of the immune response" (10). Just like muscle cells, immune cells require fuel to function. Exercise, specifically prolonged periods of intense exercise, could limit the amount of energy available for these cells and be a contributing factor to the open-window phenomenon (Simpson et al. 2020).

Carbohydrates are an essential source of fuel for high-intensity exercise and should be an important component of your nutrition intake. There is evidence to suggest that restricting carbohydrate intake could suppress your immune system. Yes, managing a healthy body weight or achieving a specific aesthetic appearance may be important goals, and restricting carbohydrate intake could play a role in those outcomes; however, when it comes to training for optimal physical performance, health should take priority over appearance. "A balanced and well-diversified diet that meets the energy demands in exercising individuals is certainly a key component to maintain immune function in response to strenuous exercise," say Peake and colleagues (2017, 1084).

To ensure that your workouts do not have a deleterious effect on your immune system, when planning your high-intensity exercise sessions, be sure to make adequate preparations for managing exercise duration, and have a postworkout snack or meal ready and available, because "postexercise immune function depression is most pronounced when the exercise is continuous, prolonged (>1.5 h), of moderate to high intensity (55-75% maximum O_2 uptake), and performed without food intake" (Gleeson 2007, 693).

Optimal Rest for Your Systems

When you are training for a specific goal, using quantitative metrics and qualitative record-keeping to track your performance can help you identify inadequate recovery and the early signs of OTS before it stops your progress and keeps you from your training objectives. So far in this book, we've identified the harmful effects of too much exercise and determined the role of recovery in a workout program. The following chapters will provide specific solutions for how to incorporate recovery strategies and techniques into your overall workout program. By the end of the book, you will know how to design workout programs structured around periods of active rest or lower-intensity exercise so that you can achieve optimal physical performance for all of your goals. In addition, you will know the benefits of many types of recovery techniques and the best times to use them. Overtraining and a lack of appropriate recovery after high-intensity workouts are the problems; the rest of this book will focus on the solutions.

4

RECOVERY METHODS

High-intensity exercise creates a physical overload on the body's systems. The purpose of the postexercise recovery period is to facilitate a rapid return to homeostasis. Rest is an essential, yet often overlooked, component of exercise. The rest period after a hard workout allows muscles to replace the glycogen and adenosine triphosphate (ATP) that fuel activity during exercise. Exercising too frequently without proper rest creates excessive overload on the metabolic pathways and does not allow enough time to replace the energy burned in a workout. However, not every workout requires a focus on recovery, especially not low- to moderate-intensity sessions that do not overstress body tissues or deplete glycogen stores.

When designing your workouts and planning your training calendar, it is important to identify specific recovery strategies that can mitigate the effects of exercise and promote optimal tissue repair and replenishment of expended energy once the workout is over. Just as an exercise program is specific to the individual, a recovery program should be designed to meet the exact needs of your schedule. If you are a busy professional and you know that certain times of the year, such as an annual meeting or budget planning, can really eat into your schedule, then knowing how to plan quick, effective workouts provides you with practical solutions that could help you reduce your overall stress load while maintaining the gains from the workouts you have been doing the rest of the year. Recovery doesn't just mean rest time; using a percussion gun to reduce muscle tension, following a high-intensity training day with a low-intensity workout, or simply going for a long walk are all strategies that could help your muscles recover from a challenging workout on the previous day so they can be ready for whatever they need to do on the following one.

Stress Requires a Specific Method of Recovery

Recovery strategies aren't just for superstar athletes. Anyone who experiences a significant amount of stress that disrupts homeostasis could benefit from strategies to minimize or mitigate the effects of that stress. In a 2017 interview on the *Joe Rogan Experience* podcast, Metallica guitarist and singer James Hetfield described how he and his bandmates have evolved their postconcert habits as they have aged past their 50s. In their younger days, the band was legendary for their postconcert entertainment; however, during the interview, Hetfield said that now, after a concert, he and his bandmates will have a kale smoothie or an organic meal and then either get a massage or be adjusted by a chiropractor (apparently, 30-plus years of banging your head has an effect on your spine). Think of postexercise recovery as a component of overall self-care. Specific techniques such as the postconcert nutrition and tissue treatment described by Hetfield could benefit anyone who experiences physical stress.

The previous chapters discussed overtraining syndrome (OTS) and how it could affect your performance and keep you from getting the results you want. This chapter will review specific strategies that could help promote a rapid return to homeostasis following a grueling workout or challenging competition or after rocking out to a stadium full of energetic fans. Whether you exercise to improve your health, to enhance your athletic performance, or just because you like the feeling of working to a point of fatigue, planning for what you do after you exercise is as important, if not more so, than planning the exercises, repetitions, and sets that make you sweat.

Workouts That Require Specific Recovery

Exercise to improve health or change the body's appearance requires a different kind of program than exercise to enhance athletic performance. However, high-intensity exercise is a component of each. High-intensity exercise can provide many benefits, but as the previous chapters have explained, too much high-intensity exercise combined with a lack of focus on the postworkout recovery phase could result in an accumulation of stress that will keep you from getting the results you want. With exercise, your body can become capable of remarkable feats; however, it is designed to operate most efficiently at homeostasis. Chronic disruption of homeostasis from excessive amounts of high-intensity exercise can contribute to OTS and a loss of physical performance.

Low- to moderate-intensity exercise that increases your breathing rate without making you out of breath requires no specific recovery strategy other than proper nutrition and a good night's sleep. However, high-intensity workouts done to lose weight, stimulate muscle growth, or prepare for athletic competition can disrupt homeostasis to the point where a specific strategy could help facilitate the return to a resting state.

Every individual responds to exercise in a different way, but in general, only exercise at the highest levels of intensity requires a specific approach to recovery. Using the 1-to-10 rating of perceived exertion (RPE) scale introduced in chapter 2, where 10 is the highest intensity possible, any workout that can be classified as 7 or higher requires a specific postexercise recovery strategy. Any workout classified as 6 or below could be considered moderate intensity or lower and would not require anything more specific than a healthy meal and a good night's sleep. Table 4.1 explains the strategy to use for different levels of workout intensity.

TABLE 4.1 Workouts That Require a Specific Recovery Strategy

RATING OF PERCEIVED EXERTION[*]	LEVEL OF INTENSITY	RECOVERY STRATEGY
1-4	Low: Breathing faster than normal, but can talk comfortably	None. Low-intensity exercise does not create a significant disruption of homeostasis. A low-intensity workout can be used the day after a high-intensity workout to promote optimal recovery.
5-6	Moderate: Breathing rate increases; can speak in short phrases but not complete sentences; difficult to maintain an ongoing conversation	Hydration, nutrition, and sleep. A well-balanced meal and a good night's sleep are the most effective recovery methods for moderate-intensity exercise.
7-10	High: Breathing is rapid; can barely speak single words	Hydration, nutrition, rest (sleep), and tissue treatment. The anaerobic metabolism required for high-intensity exercise produces metabolic by-products that are removed via the circulatory system. Elevating circulation above normal resting levels can help remove by-products and bring needed nutrients and hydration to the involved muscles.

*Measured on a scale of 1 to 10.

Plan Your Workout

Overtraining syndrome changes your body's ability to exercise, which in turn significantly affects the ability to perform at an intensity required for a specific event or competition or otherwise achieve your fitness goals. Because exercise is the primary stressor that causes OTS, changing the intensity and volume of exercise or stopping altogether is the most effective means of promoting a complete return to full homeostasis. The good news is that properly planning and designing your exercise program, combined with specific recovery strategies immediately and the day after a high-intensity workout, could significantly minimize the risk of OTS so you can maintain a high level of performance. As Bishop, Jones, and Woods (2008) note, "Recovery of muscle function is chiefly a matter of reversing the major cause of fatigue or damage" (1020).

Exercise depletes energy and damages muscle tissue; too much exercise without an appropriate approach to postexercise recovery could result in OTS. It may be more appropriate to think of OTS as an indication of being underrecovered. Athletes and fitness enthusiasts have traditionally pushed themselves to exercise harder to reach their goals, and maybe you have fallen into this trap. If enhancing athletic performance is your ultimate exercise goal, it might not be that additional set of exercises or extra training session that will help you earn your spot on the podium or crush that goal that's been eluding you. Maybe the missing ingredient is planning for *more* rest and *less* exercise so you can start your event completely rested with a full tank of gas.

Recovery Strategies

Postexercise recovery can be considered a component of self-care. Knowing the benefits of various recovery strategies and how to apply them could help reduce the cumulative effects of stress, both related and not related to exercise. In other words, when life gets hard and you're feeling stressed and overwhelmed, treating yourself to one of these methods isn't just good for your fitness, it's a benefit to your overall physical and mental health.

If exercise is a priority in your life, you have no doubt noticed a significant uptick in the various products and methods for promoting recovery. You could spend thousands of dollars on temperature-controlled mattresses and in-home massage therapy, but the most effective means of recovery—sleep and proper nutrition—often require no investment other than time. With regard to nutrition, there are many different approaches; the nutrition information provided in this book relates specifically to promoting recovery from exercise and will follow accepted guidelines from the U.S. Department of Agriculture. Proper nutrition is essential for proper recovery. If you follow a specific approach to nutrition, you may want to consult a registered dietitian-nutritionist (RDN) who could help you identify the most appropriate meal plan for your needs. Find one near you at www.eatright.org, the website for the Academy of Nutrition and Dietetics, the governing body for the RDN credential.

The No-Cost Recovery Solution

Wearing compression clothing, sitting in a cryogenic chamber, applying a percussion gun to muscles, using an infrared sauna, or getting a massage are all specific techniques that could help accelerate the recovery process. However, they can be expensive, so it is important to determine which ones are best for your needs and budget. The postexercise recovery phase is when your muscles are actually changing, which explains why so many tools have been developed to promote this process. However, the recovery method that might produce the greatest benefit is simply getting an appropriate amount of rest, either by alternating the intensity of exercise or improving the quality and quantity of your sleep. Rest is one of the most effective recovery methods and one that can be achieved by developing healthy sleep hygiene (covered in chapter 9) and alternating the intensity of workouts from one day to the next (addressed in chapter 8).

The Four Components of Recovery

Numerous methods and techniques can help promote postexercise recovery. The essential components of any recovery strategy are hydration to replace exercise-related water loss, nutrition to replace energy and promote tissue repair, rest to allow time for your physiology to completely return to homeostasis, and tissue treatment to help reduce overall tightness while enhancing circulation to remove the by-products from anaerobic metabolism. Table 4.2 describes the function of each of these strategies.

From these four general categories of recovery strategies, there are a range of methods you can use to help promote postexercise recovery (table 4.3). How these methods work and exactly when you should use them for optimal results will be addressed in the following chapters.

TABLE 4.2 Strategies That Promote Postexercise Recovery

STRATEGY	FUNCTION
Hydration	Water lost during exercise should be replaced. Blood and muscle tissue are approximately 70% water; a loss of hydration could reduce the ability to deliver energy to working muscles and affect overall performance.
Nutrition	The purpose of recovery nutrition is to replace energy spent during exercise and promote the repair of muscles damaged during exercise. Postexercise nutrition should include all macronutrients essential for refueling and repair.
Rest	Rest can be active (low-intensity activity or exercise) or passive (enjoying a television show binge on your favorite streaming platform). Rest may seem like you are not doing anything, but nothing could be further from the truth. During the postexercise rest period, your physiology will be working to prepare for the next bout of moderate- to high-intensity activity.
Tissue treatment	Tissues can be treated to remove excessive metabolites and by-products of anaerobic metabolism, which could be a component of delayed-onset muscle soreness. Tissue treatment can also be done to reduce the risk of excessive muscle tightness and adhesions between layers of muscle and connective tissue. Specific tools and techniques include percussion guns, foam rolling, kinesiology tape, massage, cupping, or temperature variations (hot or cold).

TABLE 4.3 Specific Methods to Promote Recovery From Exercise

RECOVERY METHOD	GENERAL STRATEGY	HOW IT WORKS
Passive rest (no structured, specific physical activity)	Rest	During rest, the physiological systems of the body repair themselves to replace energy in muscle cells, repair damaged tissues, and remove metabolic waste. Passive rest with minimal activity can be one of the most effective ways to completely recover from regular exercise or even the effects of overtraining syndrome.
Active rest (low-intensity exercise)	Rest	Low- to moderate-intensity mobility exercises (a rating of perceived exertion between 3-6 on a scale of 1-10) that move the body through multiple planes of motion can elevate tissue temperature and circulation, both of which help to promote a complete recovery. Low-intensity workouts allow you to move for the purpose of elevating circulation and burning calories.
Sleep	Rest	Your body produces testosterone and growth hormone, used for tissue repair, during the deep rapid-eye-movement cycles of sleep, making it important to get a full night's sleep on the days that you plan your highest-intensity workouts. If you have a busy period of work, travel, or family obligations, you should adjust your exercise program accordingly with low- to moderate-intensity workouts until you can return to normal sleep patterns that can support higher-intensity exercise.
Compression Clothing Pneumatic pressure	Tissue treatment	Whether it's from specially designed elastic clothing or cuffs that wrap the entire leg for the purpose of applying pneumatic air compression, external pressure against muscle tissue helps promote venous return of deoxygenated blood (carrying the by-products of anaerobic metabolism) to the heart and lungs. Deoxygenated blood is pumped to the lungs, where carbon dioxide is removed and freshly inspired oxygen is put in so it can be pumped to the muscles to help support the recovery process. Compression can also help reduce fatigue and delayed-onset muscle soreness.
Myofascial release Percussion gun Foam roller Rolling stick Scraping Massage therapy	Tissue treatment	Optimal recovery for the myofascial network goes beyond simply stretching and should include techniques for improving tissue extensibility (the ability of separate layers of muscle tissue to slide across one another) using percussion guns, foam rollers, rolling sticks, scrapers, or even massage from a professional therapist. The goal is to apply appropriate pressure to the muscle tissue to improve circulation and reduce the opportunity for inelastic collagen fibers to develop in stress points, which can limit tissue extensibility. Equipment for myofascial release can be affordable, making it an effective solution that can be done every evening while watching your favorite television-streaming platform.
Heat Sauna Steam room Hot tub	Tissue treatment	The heat from a sauna, steam room, or hot tub increases the body's circulation, which removes metabolic waste products such as hydrogen ions while carrying oxygen and other nutrients necessary to help repair tissue used during a workout.
Cold treatment Ice applied to wrists and neck Cold-water plunge Ice bath Cryogenic chamber	Tissue treatment	Ice baths, ice packs, cooling vests, or special chairs with pockets for ice packs are all options for applying cold treatment. One benefit of cold treatment is helping to lower the body's core temperature, which is essential when exercising in hot weather or playing in tournaments that have multiple competitions on the same day. Cold treatment can also reduce inflammation and promote healing in tissue that was used during a workout. The application of ice to a sore muscle or joint brings more blood to the area, which brings nutrients and oxygen to help promote healing.
Nutrition	Nutrition	Moderate- to high-intensity exercise depletes muscles of stored energy; the study of nutrient timing suggests that *when* nutrition is consumed relative to high-intensity exercise may be more important than *what* is consumed. After exercise, the body needs to replenish energy with carbohydrates and repair tissue with protein. A postworkout snack or drink with a proper ratio of carbohydrates to protein can help with both needs. The carbohydrates will refuel energy needs and the protein supports postexercise muscle repair. Proper timing of nutrient intake relative to exercise can promote glycogen replacement and protein resynthesis.

Budgeting for Recovery

If you are worried about how much money you may need to invest in various recovery strategies, take comfort in the fact that the most effective methods do not necessarily cost anything, but they do need a mindful approach with program design and implementation. Planning your postexercise recovery can be done for very little money. Proper nutrition and rest are two of the most effective recovery methods available. Other techniques, like the tissue treatments mentioned in table 4.3, can also help accelerate the return to homeostasis; however, it is important to know when and how to apply them so they can have the greatest possible effect. If you are a member of a full-service health club, one of the benefits is that besides having the latest exercise equipment, many offer amenities such as a hot tub, sauna, or steam room, along with equipment like foam rollers and stretching areas that can be used to facilitate the recovery process. Many health clubs even offer specific recovery rooms that include massage chairs, pressure cuffs, percussion guns, and other tools that can help members achieve optimal postexercise recovery.

Timing of Recovery

One of the most important components of a successful exercise program is the ability to be physically active every day, which is why you should begin your workout knowing exactly how you will recover once you're done sweating. There are four time periods to consider for recovery: the rest period after completing a set of an exercise (or series of exercises when circuit training) during a workout; immediately after the workout or competition is over (in the coming chapters, the terms *workout* and *training session* will refer to any type of vigorous physical activity, including competition); the day after a workout, when muscles are still in the process of repairing tissue as well as replacing energy; and long term. Any workout program should be designed to allow for periods of rest so the body has time to completely recover and be ready to go.

Within-Workout Rest

High-intensity exercise, whether metabolic conditioning or strength training, should be performed to a point of momentary fatigue, which is an indication that no more energy is immediately available in the muscle cells. Exercising to a point of fatigue necessitates a brief period, up to five minutes, immediately after the completion of one bout of exercise to allow muscle cells to regenerate ATP in order to be properly fueled for the next. The rest period immediately after completing an exercise is essential to allow muscle cells the time to regenerate and replace energy.

Case Study: Allison

Allison is a 35-year-old woman who was a scholarship runner in college and competed in cross country and middle-distance track. Allison is married, has two kids in elementary school, and works full time from home. She is still an age-group runner for both the 5K and 10K (3 mi and 6 mi); however, she hasn't pushed herself to be competitive since having her children. Now that she is 35 years old and eligible for master's-level races, Allison is training to be competitive, with a goal of finishing in the top 10 of her age group in each race. In preparation for the upcoming race season, Allison is planning both strength training workouts to improve her muscle-force output and high-intensity interval training to boost her aerobic capacity without having to train at a high volume. As a result of her renewed focus on her training, Allison is searching for solutions to improve her ability to recover after a hard run or between races.

To achieve her goal of placing in the top 10 of every race, Allison knows she will need to improve her recovery efforts so that she can increase the volume of her training. Allison has started working with an RDN who can help her develop a nutrition program that provides the appropriate level of macronutrients for her training and race needs; in addition, she has invested in a percussion gun and massage stick to help lower the risk of injury by reducing muscle tightness and improving mobility. After listening to a podcast on the performance benefits of sleep, Allison has committed to improving her sleep hygiene and has purchased compression pants to wear while sleeping. Finally, Allison wears a smartwatch, which allows her to monitor her heart rate while exercising as well as her heart-rate variability during the recovery phase after exercise.

Based on her years of experience, Allison recognizes that if she is feeling fatigued, it is better to rest a day than try to train on an empty tank; as a result, she tracks how she feels after her workouts and when she wakes up in the morning so that she knows when she can train hard and when she should take an unplanned rest day.

The Day of a High-Intensity Workout

Immediately after a high-intensity workout is over is the most important time to focus on applying specific recovery strategies. The primary goal should be to replace energy and hydration lost during exercise. The secondary objective is tissue treatment, such as using a foam roller or percussion gun or sitting in a sauna or cold bath to promote the mechanical repair process. Postexercise nutrition, tissue treatment, and rest are all important components of recovery immediately after a workout. Chapter 6 will address specific methods and strategies you can use to promote a return to homeostasis once a workout is complete.

The Day After a High-Intensity Workout

A low-intensity bodyweight workout to emphasize mobility, tissue treatment with a percussion gun followed by a long walk, or low-intensity strength training to move joints through their structural range of motion while elevating circulation are among strategies that could be used to promote recovery the day after a high-intensity workout. Rest is an essential component of recovery, but low-intensity exercise can provide important benefits that help promote a complete return to homeostasis. Chapter 7 explains the key components of recovery the day after a hard workout.

Planning Workouts for Long-Term Success

High-intensity exercise is popular because it delivers results for both aesthetic and health goals, and in limited amounts, it *is* good for you; however, the challenge is that the same high-intensity workouts that deliver results could also cause soreness and limit your ability to exercise the following day. In addition, too many high-intensity workouts without the proper time for rest and recovery could result in OTS. Therefore, to achieve optimal results, it is important to design a workout program that alternates between low-, moderate-, and high-intensity exercise. Chapter 8 explains how to create a periodized plan for yourself that alternates between low-, moderate-, and high-intensity workouts. In addition, you will learn specific strategies and healthy habits that can help you avoid OTS so you can achieve and sustain an optimal state of fitness.

Planning for Recovery

The time after exercise is when your physiology is adapting to the demands imposed during the workout, and specific strategies can facilitate a rapid return to homeostasis so that your muscles can properly rest, refuel, rehydrate, and repair before the next competition or training session. No matter what your specific goals are, when designing an exercise program, consider the volume of high-intensity exercise and plan appropriate strategies to promote optimal recovery between the challenging workouts that create the changes you want to make to your body. If your performance is important to you, then you need to make recovery a consistent habit by making smart choices with nutrition, getting good sleep, making time for low-intensity workouts, and applying treatment strategies to your muscle and connective tissues after every challenging workout or whenever you may be feeling any excessive tightness or stiffness. The evidence strongly suggests that spending as much time programming your recovery as you do your workouts could help you crush your training goals.

5

FASCIA AND FOAM ROLLING

Picture a young boy, about five or six years old, and imagine that he is set free on a playground. What would you see? A little boy at play would no doubt be a bundle of energy, climbing, jumping, running, and moving in all directions at various speeds. Now picture an older man in his 70s trying to navigate a busy city sidewalk. How would an older man move differently than a young boy? Being wary of having to navigate around distractions such as other walkers, the older man would probably move slower, be more cautious, and have a limited range of motion compared with the boy. If they have the same basic structure and anatomy, why would the two move so differently?

The answer comes down to the myofascial network and its ability to control forces moving through the body at all velocities and in all directions. Excessive amounts of repetitive movements combined with poor hydration and inadequate tissue treatment for the fascia could result in a loss of tissue elasticity and joint mobility. However, proper care and treatment of your myofascial network via nutrition, hydration, and tissue-treatment strategies during the recovery phase of exercise could help you to maintain elasticity similar to the young boy's throughout your life span. Making time for proper care of your tissues after high-intensity exercise could allow you to maintain energy and movement skills even in the later years of your life, so this should be an essential component of your overall fitness program. (To learn more about how exercise can slow aging, refer to *Ageless Intensity: High-Intensity Workouts to Slow the Aging Process.*)

Foam rolling can help alleviate muscle tightness while promoting optimal circulation, making it a mode of recovery-promoting exercise that could be done daily. Tissue treatment is an important component of recovery because every muscle is connected to another; if one set of muscles is affected by overuse, it will influence how surrounding muscles perform and function. Effective recovery workouts that involve all muscles working together to promote whole-body movement patterns can elevate the systemic circulation that promotes tissue repair. To be most effective, some recovery strategies, such as tissue treatment, should be applied daily; this chapter addresses the mechanical functions of fascia to explain why it requires proper treatment after high-intensity exercise. This knowledge will allow you to take better care of your body, which, in turn, will allow your body to take better care of you.

Myofascial Network

If you have been doing workouts that focus on only one body part or muscle group at a time, you may want to reconsider, especially if you are training for a specific sport. When we move, our brains do not consciously think about the actions individual muscles perform; instead, the brain identifies a movement we need to execute, and our muscles react according to this intention.

Muscle fibers contain motor units, which convert signals from the central nervous system into muscle contractions and compose the contractile element that generates the forces to produce movement. Elastic fascia and connective tissues surround every individual muscle fiber, connecting muscles to one another and to skeletal structures; these tissues distribute the forces produced by the contractile element throughout the body.

Two Components of Muscle

The two specific components of skeletal muscle tissue are striated muscle, composed of the contractile element responsible for producing movement, and the elastic fascia and connective tissues interwoven between the various layers of muscle. Striated skeletal muscle is enveloped by fascia and other connective tissues, and when healthy, the entire structure can be pliable, easily allowing surrounding joints to move unrestricted through their structural ranges of motion (Myers 2020; Schleip 2015).

A practical definition of *fascia*, established by delegates of the first Fascia Research Congress in 2007, is "all collagenous fibrous connective tissues that can be seen as elements of a body-wide tensional force transmission network" (Schleip 2015, 3). In this chapter, the term *fascia* will be used to represent all elastic connective tissues that surround every individual muscle fiber, attach different muscles to one another, and connect muscles to bones. Research suggests that noncontractile connective tissue is the richest sensory organ in the human body, containing up to 10 times as many free nerve endings as the contractile element (Schleip et al. 2012). Adhesions in fascia could stimulate nociceptors, the sensory neurons that send pain signals to the brain; the purpose of tissue-treatment strategies is to reduce stress in the fascia in order to minimize discomfort by reducing pressure on the nerve endings that sense pain while ensuring the ability of layers of muscle tissue to slide across one another to generate force.

The entire myofascial network is a wholly integrated system responsible for establishing a constant equilibrium of forces within your body. This means that during a high-intensity workout, most of your muscles are involved in some way or another, which helps to explain the overall soreness felt the following day. It is often the large, prime-mover muscles that perform a majority of the work, and as a result, they require most of the attention for tissue treatment.

Contractile Element

The fascia, or connective tissue, which surrounds each layer of the contractile element is itself organized into different components (figure 5.1):

- the endomysium, the connective tissue around an individual myofibril (muscle fiber);

- the perimysium, the layer of connective tissue around a fascicle (bundle of muscle fibers); and
- the epimysium, the outermost layer of connective tissue around an entire muscle or collection of fascicles.

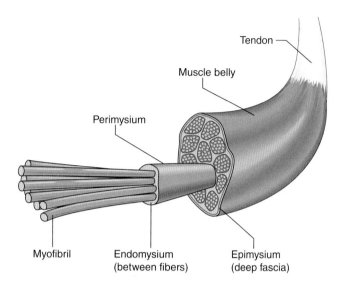

FIGURE 5.1 Muscle contains different layers of fibers separated by connective tissue; collagen can bind between the layers, creating adhesions that can impede muscle function and reduce mobility.

Reprinted by permission from P.A. Houglum, K.L. Boyle-Walker, and D.E. Houglum, *Rehabilitation of Musculoskeletal Injuries* (Champaign, IL: Human Kinetics, 2023), 386.

The contractile element produces muscle contractions that are generally categorized as follows (figure 5.2):

- *Eccentric: a lengthening action where the resistive force is overcoming the muscular force.* Eccentric muscle actions cause significant amounts of force as muscle fibers slide against one another; workouts that feature high eccentric loads could cause significant amounts of delayed-onset muscle soreness.
- *Concentric: a shortening action where the muscular force is overcoming the resistive force.* The force for a concentric muscle action starts with the contractile element but is distributed through the fascial network to involve surrounding muscles and tissues.
- *Isometric: an action where the muscle fibers are shortening but no joint motion occurs.* During explosive plyometric muscle actions, the muscle fibers will remain in an isometric contraction to place tension on the elastic fascia; the greater the amount of force created during an isometric contraction, the greater the force distributed to the fascia and elastic connective tissues.

The contractile element of your muscular system contains both type I muscle fibers, the cells of which rely on aerobic metabolism of free fatty acids for adenosine triphosphate (ATP), and type II fibers, the cells of which produce energy from glycogen, either with or without oxygen. The larger type II muscle fibers are the component of the contractile element that generates the force for move-

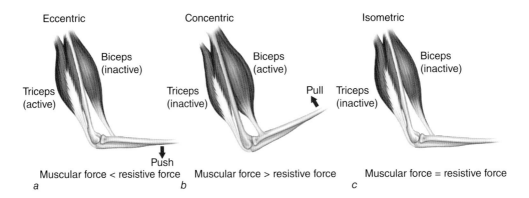

FIGURE 5.2 The three different types of muscle contractions: *(a)* eccentric, *(b)* concentric, and *(c)* isometric. Because there is significant tension between muscle fibers during eccentric contractions, they can result in the greatest amount of muscle damage.

Reprinted by permission from F. Naclerio and J. Moody, "Resistance Training," in *EuropeActive's Foundations for Exercise Professionals*, edited by T. Rieger, F. Naclerio, A. Jiménez, and J. Moody (Champaign, IL: Human Kinetics, 2015), 66.

ment, and when ATP is metabolized anaerobically, there is a rapid buildup of metabolic by-products, which could result in fatigue and delayed-onset muscle soreness the day after a hard workout unless the appropriate tissue-treatment strategies are applied. On the day of a hard workout, select a specific tissue-repair strategy—myofascial release, temperature treatment, or compression clothing—to accompany rehydration, proper nutrition, and a good night's sleep for an optimal postworkout recovery. Low-intensity exercise that elevates circulation is an effective strategy the day after a workout because it can help flush the remaining metabolic by-products from the muscle tissue.

Daily tissue treatment is important because without proper care, your fascia could develop adhesions, collections of collagen proteins along specific lines of stress that restrict the ability of layers of tissue to slide over one another during movement. Referred to as Davis' law, when collagen cells bind along the lines of stress, they could cause the muscle fibers to stick together, resulting in an adhesion that restricts the ability of muscle tissue to generate and distribute force. Repetitive movements, such as running or cycling for long distances, could cause such adhesions, or knots (MacDonald, Penney, et al. 2013).

Mechanical Properties of Fascia

As a form of connective tissue, fascia provides protection, support, and structure to the contractile element of muscle tissue and is an important component of the tissues that make up the tendons, which attach muscles to bone; the ligaments, which connect one bone to another; and the periosteum, which covers the surface of a bone (Schleip 2017). (Although bone is often perceived as a solid structure, it is a collagen-based, living tissue that is malleable and capable of adapting to mechanical forces, just like other tissues.) During human movement, as fascia is lengthened, it stores mechanical potential energy that is released during the shortening phase of muscle action. It is estimated that fascia can return approximately 90 percent of energy during many movement patterns; however, when fascia becomes tight or experiences a restriction that limits its ability to return to its original position after lengthening, this could change how a nearby joint functions (Earls 2014). Specific postexercise tissue-treatment strategies could help improve circulation to remove metabolic by-products and replace intracellular energy stores while ensuring that fascia maintains the mechanical properties to lengthen and shorten in response to applied forces.

Some other important facts about fascia include the following (Schleip 2015):

- The average body contains between 40 and 51 pounds (18 to 23 kg) of fascia.
- Fascia responds to stress and strain and is constantly generating cells for repairing or building new tissue.
- As much as 40 percent of muscle force is generated by the mechanical efforts of fascia.

There are two specific components of fascia: the individual protein fibers of collagen and elastin and the extracellular matrix (ECM) (figure 5.3*a*), containing fibroblasts—individual cells of fibrous connective tissue and ground substance (figure 5.3*b*), where proteoglycans hold on to water. All cells are formed within this fluid that plays in integral role in creating the structure of the body. The ECM surrounds individual muscle and fascia fibers like a soft, coarse mesh that contains nerve endings, sensory neurons, and glands responsible for producing specific hormones (Schleip 2017). Collagen is a structural protein bound in a triple-helix formation to give it rigidity, which is why it is used as a building block for many tissues in the body (figure 5.3*c*). Fascia is mostly collagen but also contains elastin, a protein that lengthens in response to a tensile (lengthening) force and returns to the original resting position once the force is removed. Collagen and elastin contain fibroblasts, which are individual cells produced in response to mechanical forces and function as the construction workers of the body because they can repair damaged tissue or build new tissue, including collagen, in response to a mechanical stress (Myers 2020).

How Adhesions Happen

Ground substance is a collection of individual collagen molecules that compose the ECM surrounding individual muscle fibers. During normal movement and activity, collagen will be produced parallel to muscle fibers to provide structure and elasticity, helping the tissue to be more resilient and less susceptible to a strain injury. The ECM is a viscous fluid that can reduce friction as individual muscle fibers slide against one another. When muscle tissue is moved frequently, the ECM increases temperature and becomes more gel-like, reducing friction and allowing easier movement between individual fibers. However, a combination of dehydration and lack of movement can cause the ECM to become stickier, limiting the ability of fibers to slide against one another. This explains an additional benefit of rehydrating immediately after a hard workout; it allows the layers of your muscles to slide over one another more easily to reduce the risk of developing adhesions. When muscle fibers remain inactive for an extended length of time, the collagen molecules of the ECM could actually bind together for stability, which creates the adhesions between the various layers of muscle that ultimately become painful trigger points (Schleip 2015). When adhesions form, they could cause a muscle to remain in a shortened position, which restricts its ability to allow movement at a joint; using a foam roller, percussion gun, or other type of tissue treatment after you have finished a high-intensity workout, combined with proper rehydration to increase intracellular fluid levels, could reduce the risk of developing adhesions, allowing your muscles to function at their optimal level of performance.

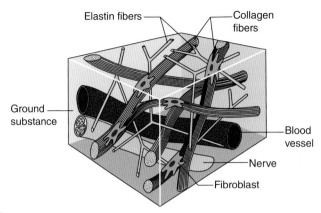

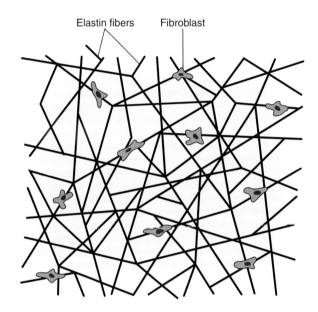

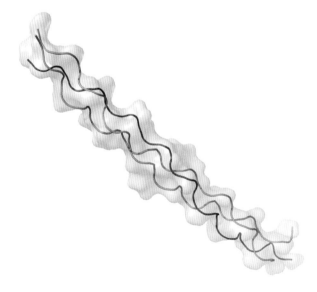

FIGURE 5.3 *(a)* The components of the extracellular matrix, *(b)* ground substance, and *(c)* collagen. A lack of proper hydration can reduce the ability of fibers to slide against one another and cause adhesions that limit mobility.

(For *a* and *b*) Reprinted by permission from J. Watkins, *Structure and Function of the Musculoskeletal System,* 2nd ed. (Champaign, IL: Human Kinetics, 2010), 67.

The natural inflammation that occurs during the tissue-repair process, combined with a lack of movement after an exercise session, could be another cause of muscle adhesions. Exercise-induced muscle damage signals the repair process. This is when new collagen molecules are formed to help repair and strengthen tissue; if tissue is not moved, the collagen could bind between layers of muscle (figure 5.4). Muscle damage can change the firing patterns of the motor units responsible for muscle contractions and change the sequence in which muscles are recruited and engaged to produce a movement (MacDonald, Penney et al. 2013). Myofascial release can help minimize the risk that the new collagen will form adhesions between layers and can possibly reduce the length of time it takes to completely return to homeostasis.

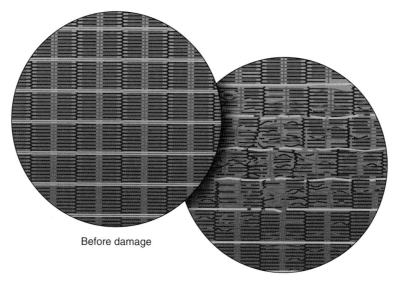

Before damage

Damaged muscle fibers

FIGURE 5.4   High-intensity exercise can damage muscle cells; this type of disruption requires an appropriate amount of recovery so muscles can achieve optimal performance.

Reprinted by permission from B. Murray and W.L. Kenney, *Practical Guide to Exercise Physiology* (Champaign, IL: Human Kinetics, 2016), 18.

Biotensegrity and the Human Body

At the very beginning of your life, you were a single-cell organism that experienced rapid growth via cell division during the gestation period. By the time you were born, all cells and bodily tissues, specifically muscle and fascia, were connected to create an entirely integrated system (Myers 2020; Schultz and Feitis 1996). Tensegrity is a combination of tension and integrity and is an architectural term used to describe a structure that is self-supporting through a combination of tensile (lengthening) and compressive (shortening) forces. Because the myofascial system is designed to balance the forces of compression and tension, the term *biotensegrity* describes the body's natural structural tendency to balance the mechanical forces created by high-intensity muscle contractions (Galli et al. 2005; Ingber 2003; Myers 2020). Although the body is designed to mitigate these forces, the stress can still accumulate and change the function of both muscles and fascia, especially when combined with the by-products from anaerobic metabolism. Making tissue treatment a daily habit is an important component of your overall training strategy because it could help to promote recovery and ensure that your tissues remain capable of functioning at an optimal level of performance.

Although traditional anatomy teaches that the skeletal system provides the structure for how the body moves, applying the biotensegrity model of movement, it is more accurate to say that the bones float within a three-dimensional matrix of both muscle and connective tissue, making proper tissue treatment essential for ensuring that the system functions to the best of its ability (Myers 2020). Fascia is a living tissue that maintains a constant balance between the synthesis of new cells and the remodeling of existing cells in response to external and internal forces. The primary regulators of tensegrity—tension and compression—influence a cell's biochemical response to stress; the biotensegrity model of human anatomy has been shown to accurately predict mechanical behaviors of human cells (Ingber 2003, 2004).

Applying the biotensegrity model to the human body explains how forces introduced at one point in a structure will be transmitted throughout the entire system. As a result, for most exercises, when you are lifting a weight, it is not just the immediate muscles that do the work; a wide network of muscles contributes and shares in the force production, which explains why you might experience soreness throughout your entire body the day after a hard, full-body workout. This also explains why a full-body workout of low-intensity mobility exercises can feel so good the day after a hard workout; as you move through different patterns and planes of motion, the entire myofascial network experiences elevated temperatures and circulation, which help to reduce any feelings of soreness or fatigue.

How Force Builds Fascia

Mechanotransduction is the word used to describe how mechanical force creates chemical change in the human body. More specifically, mechanical forces affecting the body signal the production of satellite cells, which become the fibroblasts that repair damaged tissues, both with proteins that make up individual muscle fibers and collagen that becomes a component of elastic connective tissues. Fibroblasts can repair damaged muscle fibers in addition to creating stronger connective tissues capable of withstanding greater levels of mechanical force. This explains why moving your body multidirectionally with low-intensity resistance is an effective strategy the day after a hard workout; it is stimulating the production of fibroblasts to increase the strength and resilience of your fascia and elastic connective tissues. Lengthening fascia and elastic connective tissues under resistance applies tensile forces that stimulate the production of new fibroblasts for creating the collagen fibers, which ultimately help the elastic connective tissues become stronger and more resistant to injury (Schleip 2015).

Mechanical Energy

Muscles use two types of energy to generate movement: chemical energy from ATP, metabolized from the macronutrients in the diet; and elastic mechanical energy, released as the result of muscles being rapidly lengthened before quickly transitioning to the shortening phase of muscle action. During an explosive muscle action, the contractile element of muscle fibers remains in a shortened position, which then increases tension on the elastic fascia. When external forces, created by the combination of gravity and external loads, are applied to the myofascial network, the fibers of the contractile element can shorten and create tension, while the surrounding viscoelastic noncontractile component lengthens (Myers 2020; Verkoshansky and Siff 2009).

When the surrounding fascia is lengthened, it is experiencing a tensile force that stores elastic mechanical energy, which is then released as the muscle transitions to the shortening phase; this is known as the stretch–shorten cycle of muscle action. The stretch–shorten cycle describes how the myofascial network functions as a wholly integrated mechanical system using the competing forces of tension and compression responsible for storing and releasing mechanical energy. Increasing the ability of the contractile element to maintain force while shortened, combined with enhancing the ability of the elastic tissues to lengthen and shorten, can increase overall levels of force production during athletic movements.

Both forms of energy production require appropriate strategies to ensure an optimal recovery. Nutrition supplies the carbohydrates, fats, and proteins used to replace energy, promote hormone production, and repair tissues, respectively, whereas tissue-treatment strategies can help promote circulation to remove metabolic by-products and promote the healing process for the tissues involved with producing mechanical energy. Tissue treatment in the 24 hours after exercise is critical for optimizing the ability to generate mechanical energy, because if adhesions form between layers of muscle fibers or fascia, it could affect the ability of muscles to properly lengthen and shorten to generate force.

An adhesion can occur in a muscle if fibroblasts collect to repair or strengthen a spot that experiences abnormal stress. Think of fibroblasts as acting like a patch on the rubber inner tube of a bicycle tire; you can glue a patch on the tube to stop the leak of air, but it will restrict that area's ability to expand at the same rate as the rest of the inner tube. Fibroblasts function to strengthen the area immediately around damaged tissue, but the fibers could form perpendicular to the existing fibers, which can change the ability of the tissue to lengthen and shorten. Foam rolling on a consistent basis can help ensure that when fibroblasts are produced, they end up forming muscle fibers that are parallel to the existing ones.

The myofascial network is so efficient at transferring force from one section to another that a muscle does not have to cross a joint to create movement at that joint. For example, the soleus attaches to the top of the tibia bone of the lower leg and does not cross the knee; when you are walking forward and your right leg is on the ground, as the body passes over your right foot, the right soleus controls forward motion of the tibia (Neumann 2010). If repetitive stress from high-intensity exercise causes an adhesion in the soleus, it could change how it functions, which in turn could change the motion of the ankle or knee joints. In this case, on the day after a hard workout or competition, tissue treatment of the soleus, which can include foam rolling on the muscle followed by low-intensity, multiplanar movement patterns, could help promote the recovery process while applying minimal forces to the tissues.

How Muscle Tightness Affects Your Body

In healthy, functional muscle, the layers of tissue slide against one another with minimal restrictions. Adhesions formed by collagen binding between layers of muscle can limit tissue extensibility and significantly reduce joint motion. If a muscle on one side of a joint is held in a shortened position, it can send an inhibitory signal, causing tissue on the other side of the joint to lengthen. This creates an imbalance of forces around a particular joint, which can change both its structure and function. When adhesions form, they can cause a muscle to remain in a shortened position, which then restricts its ability to lengthen and allow movement at a joint. Changes in muscle length and joint structure can restrict normal movement patterns and cause injury in active individuals. Another factor affecting the risk of adhesions is hydration level; if tissues experience a combination of dehydration and lack of movement, then the ECM can become stickier, limiting the ability of fibers to slide against one another; when fibers remain inactive for a period of time, the collagen molecules of the ECM bind together for stability, which can create an adhesion between the various layers of muscle (Schleip 2015).

Scar tissue is an example of how collagen produced by the ECM binds together to help a tissue regain its structure after an injury. Once a scar is formed, it can limit the ability of the tissue to move through its normal range of motion, which then affects normal joint function. During traditional massage, therapists use their hands to place pressure directly on sheaths of muscle to break up collagen adhesions and realign the tissue so the layers are able to slide against one another without any restrictions. Breaking up adhesions can help reduce muscle tightness and improve a joint's range of motion; however, unless your last name is Buffett, Zuckerberg, or Gates, receiving a massage after every hard workout could be prohibitively expensive, which is why tools like foam rollers, massage sticks, and percussion guns become so important in your exercise tool box; each one allows you to give yourself the benefits of a massage without having to pay for a live-in therapist. Exercise stimulates the production of collagen to provide structural support to tissues, making them more resilient and less susceptible to a strain injury; strength training exercises that move your body through multiple planes of motion can help produce collagen that makes fascia capable of withstanding multidirectional strains (Myers 2020). Fibroblasts are produced after a hard workout to repair tissue; using a foam roller combined with a low-intensity mobility workout could help to strengthen tissue while reducing the risk of developing adhesions, which ultimately promotes recovery while maintaining optimal joint motion.

Maintaining Healthy Muscle Tissue

In healthy muscle tissue, the fascia should be hydrated sufficiently to allow the layers of muscle to slide against one another with minimal restrictions; however, adhesions can impede this movement. Changes in muscle length and joint structure can restrict normal movement patterns and can be a cause of injury for active individuals, which is why tissue-treatment strategies are so important during the postworkout recovery phase. Think of a repetitive motion such as cycling; after miles of pedaling, your calves and hip flexors have experienced a tremendous amount of mechanical stress, and the glycogen stored in muscle cells has been depleted. Applying the right tissue treatment could help the fibers heal more quickly while removing metabolic by-products and increasing circulation to help replace carbohydrate stores.

Rehydrating immediately after a workout can also ensure that the ECM remains properly lubricated to allow the layers of muscle and tissue to slide over one another. Your body is designed to be as mechanically efficient as possible and will move in the path of least resistance; however, if a mobile joint does not allow freedom for uninhibited movement, then a nearby stable joint will have to allow that motion to occur. When the stability and mobility relationships between joints become altered, the extensibility of the surrounding muscle and connective tissue also changes, affecting the ability to perform and control efficient movement patterns (Cook 2010).

The Science of Foam Rolling

The use of foam rollers is the most affordable and accessible method of self-myofascial release (SMR), the technique of using applied pressure to reduce overall tightness and increase a muscle's resting length. Foam rollers are very affordable and can be purchased at most sporting goods stores or big-box retailers with a fitness aisle; in addition, they are a standard item in most modern fitness facilities around the world.

The pressure and motion of a muscle moving on a foam roller helps to break up adhesions and realign muscle tissue so it can function normally (Mauntel, Clark, and Padua 2014). In general, foam rollers provide the greatest response when you place a muscle directly on the roller and move in a steady, rhythmic pace to apply pressure to the underlying tissues. As you are foam rolling, you should feel mild discomfort as the muscle tension is reduced; however, if you feel a tight spot of acute soreness, that indicates a trigger point where collagen is starting to form in response to mechanical forces. Maintain pressure as you roll over the trigger point for 30 to 60 seconds to reduce tightness and stimulate blood flow.

There are two prevailing theories on why foam rolling works to alleviate muscle tightness. These are discussed in the following sections.

Foam Rolling and Autogenic Inhibition

The first hypothesis on how foam rolling works is that it creates length change. This theory is based on the principle of autogenic inhibition, which happens when intrinsic sensory receptors—the Golgi tendon organs (GTOs) and muscle spindles—identify changes within muscle tissue. The GTOs sense tension placed on a muscle, whereas the spindles identify length change and the rate of change within a particular muscle. Autogenic inhibition is the response that occurs; as a muscle is placed under tension, the GTOs sense the tension and send a signal to the spindles to allow the muscle to lengthen (figure 5.5). In the case of foam rolling, the pressure of the foam roller on the muscle increases tension on the muscle fibers, signaling the GTOs to allow the muscle spindles and fibers to lengthen. This is also the basic physiological mechanism for how static stretching creates length change in muscles; acute tension in the muscle leads to a neurological signal that allows the muscle to lengthen (Mauntel, Clark, and Padua 2014; Mohr, Long, and Goad 2014).

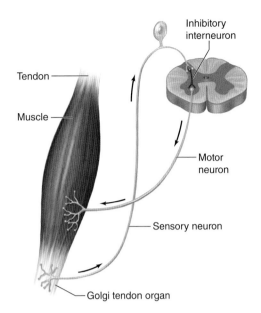

FIGURE 5.5 Pressure on muscle fibers can cause the Golgi tendon organs (GTOs) to inhibit and turn off muscle fibers so they can reduce tension, lengthen, and allow for optimal mobility.

Reprinted by permission from D. Hansen and S. Kennelly, *Plyometric Anatomy* (Champaign, IL: Human Kinetics, 2017), 6.

Foam Rolling and Muscle Temperature

The second hypothesis for how SMR with foam rolling works is that it increases the internal muscle temperature. Pressing muscle and connective tissue against a foam roller creates friction between the roller and the involved muscle, and this elevated heat causes the tissue to become more gel-like, allowing it to be more pliable. Once tissue has greater extensibility, it is easier to lengthen, allowing surrounding joints to achieve a complete range of motion free from restrictions (Healey et al. 2013; MacDonald, Button, et al. 2014; Mauntel, Clark, and Padua 2014).

It is not 100 percent clear which theory is responsible for the outcome, but myofascial foam rolling has been shown to reduce muscle tightness and increase muscle length.

Benefits of Foam Rollers

Whether it's the hands of a trained massage therapist, the rapid impacts from a percussion gun, or the pressure from a massage stick or foam roller, when a mechanical force is applied to muscle tissue, it can increase the heat of the tissue while stimulating the GTOs, both of which allow the muscle fibers to lengthen and relax. Since the early 2000s, foam rollers have become standard equipment in fitness facilities because they are effective for reducing muscle tightness. Making foam rolling a consistent part of your recovery process can help to reduce muscle tension and improve circulation, both of which will allow you to perform your best during the next hard training session or competition.

Foam rollers are very affordable, easy to use, and can help provide an immediate reduction in tightness and improvement in muscle length. One possible downside of using foam rollers is that the amount of pressure required to break up an adhesion could be uncomfortable or even painful, and this does take some getting used to; however, keep in mind that the soreness indicates muscle tension, so it is important to work through the discomfort to maintain pressure on the sore spots. The evidence observed in the scientific literature suggests that using a foam roller for myofascial release may provide the following benefits (Healey et al. 2013; MacDonald, Button, et al. 2014; Mauntel, Clark, and Padua 2014; Shah and Bhalara 2012):

- Reduced tissue tension, allowing muscles to increase joint range of motion
- Reduced risk of developing adhesions that result from collagen binding between layers of muscle tissue
- Reduced soreness after an exercise session, allowing recovery in a shorter period of time
- Promotion of a feeling of relaxation after a workout, an important psychological benefit

Benefits of Myofascial Release

The pressure and motion of a muscle moving on a foam roller can help break up adhesions and realign muscle tissue to be able to function normally (Mauntel, Clark, and Padua 2014). In general, foam rollers provide the greatest response when you place your muscle directly on top of the roller while moving slowly and rhythmically to apply pressure to the underlying tissues.

MacDonald, Button, and colleagues (2014) conducted a study with two groups: One used a foam roller after exercise to help reduce muscle tension and the other did not. Their observation was that the foam-rolling group experienced peak muscle soreness 24 hours after a workout, while the control group that did not use a foam roller experienced muscle soreness up to 48 hours after a workout. If using a foam roller can help reduce soreness and shorten the recovery time after a workout, it could allow you to increase your training volume to maximize results. In another study on the use of foam rolling for recovery, Healey and colleagues (2013, 61) observed, "Postexercise fatigue after foam rolling was significantly less . . . the reduced feeling of fatigue may allow participants to extend acute workout time and volume, which can lead to chronic performance enhancements."

In a review of the research literature on the use of foam rolling for myofascial release, Mauntel, Clark, and Padua (2014) found that applying foam rolling as a component of a warm-up can help reduce muscle tension without limiting a muscle's ability to produce force. A reduction in muscle tension can help improve joint function, allowing optimal movement efficiency and enhanced muscle performance, both of which can help reduce the risk of injury during exercise; the purpose of the review was to identify best practices for using foam rolling for SMR. Mauntel, Clark, and Padua observed that gains in joint range of motion (ROM) occurred after only 20 seconds of treatment, with more consistent results being demonstrated after 90 seconds to 3 minutes of treatment. "The findings of this study indicate that myofascial release therapies are effective in restoring and increasing ROM, without having a detrimental effect on muscular activity or performance," they reported (195-96).

Myofascial Release Tools

The first rollers developed for myofascial release were made of soft foam that would lose density and shape the more they were used. As foam rolling has become an accepted fitness practice, a wide variety of rollers have been created, each one offering specific types of benefits. A foam roller is not the only tool that provides these benefits; massage sticks and percussion guns are two other tools for applying pressure to muscle to stimulate autogenic inhibition or to increase tissue temperature. If you want to focus on a specific area of tightness or trigger point, a percussion gun or massage stick would be a better option. The two theories above that explain how foam rollers work for SMR also describe how the forces applied by a percussion gun or massage stick could help to reduce tightness and enhance blood flow. In addition, the pressure of the gun on muscle tissue can stimulate circulation to bring in additional oxygen and nutrients for tissue repair. Table 5.1 describes different types of tools and their respective uses.

Foam Roller Strategies

The natural inflammation that occurs during the tissue-repair process, combined with a lack of movement after a hard exercise session, could cause muscle adhesions, making the use of a foam roller a daily requirement during high-intensity phases of training. Exercise-induced muscle damage signals the repair process when new collagen molecules are formed to help repair and strengthen tissue; if tissue is not moved, collagen could bind between layers of muscle. Muscle damage can change the firing patterns of the motor units responsible for muscle contractions as well as the sequence in which muscles are recruited and engaged to produce a movement (MacDonald, Penney, et al. 2013). Using a foam roller can help minimize the risk that new collagen will form adhesions between layers and may possibly increase the speed of postexercise recovery.

An important benefit of foam rolling is that using a foam roller for myofascial release during a warm-up may help reduce tension while elevating temperature in muscle and fascia (Healey et al. 2013). When using a foam roller during a warm-up for a normal workout, it is important to use it for only a brief period to elevate tissue temperature and reduce tension; applying pressure from a foam roller for an extended time could desensitize the muscle, affecting its ability to contract during the workout. Think of it this way: You would not want a deep-tissue massage before a workout because it would relax a muscle and limit its ability to produce force. The same is true with a foam roller; too much pressure could reduce the effectiveness of the warm-up. However, the reason why too much foam rolling is dangerous before high-intensity exercise is exactly why it is beneficial after a workout; using the roller for an extended period of time reduces tension and feels very similar to a massage. Limit your use of a foam roller before a workout, but as a component of your recovery program, feel free to use it after the workout for as long as you feel comfortable.

The day after a hard workout, using a foam roller for myofascial release can help reduce muscle tension to increase muscle length, but this is a short-term change in the architecture of the tissue. For the best results, once myofascial release has been completed and tissues are lengthened, it is important to move through a range of motion to ensure that the involved muscles can control the change in extensibility and length. This explains why combining tissue treatment with a mobility workout is such an effective recovery strategy the day after a hard workout.

TABLE 5.1 Types of SMR Tools and Their Benefits

TYPE	DESCRIPTION	ADVANTAGES	DISADVANTAGES
Soft core foam roller	A roller made of soft foam that is easy to compress, placing less force directly on the muscle	The pliable surface allows greater contact with muscle tissue May be a more comfortable option when first introducing clients to foam rolling	Repeated use over time can cause foam to change shape and become compressed, reducing the effectiveness May not apply enough force to extremely active and fit individuals
Hard core foam roller	A foam roller with an outer surface of foam and an inner core made from hard plastic	Maintains shape over repeated uses Can apply a significant amount of pressure to the contact area of the muscle	May apply too much pressure and be uncomfortable for some individuals
High-density foam roller	A roller made from a specific type of dense foam or hard rubber that is resistant to compression (the roller pictured has a hard core and a dense surface for optimal pressure on the tissues)	The density of the foam roller allows greater pressure to be placed on areas of adhesion and tightness The thicker foam allows the roller to maintain its shape for a longer period An option for individuals who may not experience benefits of a soft roller but are not yet ready for a roller with a hard inner surface	May be too dense and cause discomfort for certain individuals
Foam rollers with patterns or grooves	Rollers with specific patterns or grooves that place pressure on different parts of a muscle	Patterns in the surface allow the roller to put different amounts of pressure on the muscle, which has been theorized to promote circulation	Depending on the type of roller, the patterning could cause increased pressure in certain areas, leading to discomfort
Balls	Alternative option to rollers; the ball shape allows pressure to be focused on specific areas; like foam rollers, balls can come in a variety of sizes and densities; many companies make specific self-myofascial release balls, but almost any type of ball, such as a golf, tennis, lacrosse, or inflatable ball, can be used	The density and size of the ball allows pressure to be placed directly on specific areas of the muscle	The surface of the ball may be difficult to adjust to a targeted area of adhesion Certain balls may be too dense and cause discomfort or pain
Rolling sticks	Alternative option to rollers; hand-held devices that can be used to apply pressure and create friction directly on adhesions and areas of tightness	Allow force to be applied directly to an adhesion or area of discomfort	Can be hard to use on certain areas of the body

FOAM ROLLER

Foam Roller Strategies

When using a foam roller for myofascial release, move at a consistent tempo of approximately one inch (2.54 cm) per second while remaining on areas of tension for up to 90 seconds to allow the tissue to relax and lengthen. When foam rolling immediately before a workout, one set of approximately 30 seconds could help to prepare for activity by increasing tissue temperature. When foam rolling after a hard workout, whether immediately after or the day after, using the roller for a longer period of time (and up to 3 sets) will cause the muscles to relax and lengthen while promoting blood flow. Perform all the movements below in sequence.

Muscles	Duration	Sets
Calves	45-60 seconds each side	1-3
Hamstrings and adductors	45-60 seconds each side	1-3
Quadriceps and hip flexors	45-60 seconds each side	1-3
Lateral quadriceps and iliotibial band	45-60 seconds each side	1-3
Latissimus dorsi	45-60 seconds each side	1-3
Lower and middle back	45-60 seconds each side	1-3

Calves

Benefits

The calf muscles are always working. When they become too tight, they can affect mobility at the ankle, which in turn can change how the hip functions. Using a foam roller can help reduce tightness to allow the ankle to have greater mobility, especially when it is on the ground during the midstance phase of the gait. Because SMR can help ensure optimal mobility of the ankle, it is a great tool to use both before and after running workouts.

Instructions

1. Sit with your legs directly in front of you and your hands under your shoulders. Keep your spine long and straight.
2. Place your left calf on top of the foam roller and bend your right knee to place your right foot flat on the ground.
3. Move forward and backward with your left calf to find a spot that is tight or tender (this tender spot is where bundles of muscle fibers have become tight; you will know it when you feel it).
4. Once you find the tender spot, roll your foot to point toward the midline of the body, then rotate it to point away from the midline of the body. After 15 to 20 seconds of rolling, move to another tight spot and repeat for 45 to 60 seconds per tender spot before switching legs. Spend the same amount of time on both legs.

Correct Your Form

If your wrists fatigue from holding yourself off the ground, or if the tightness in the calf causes too much soreness, you can stay seated on the ground.

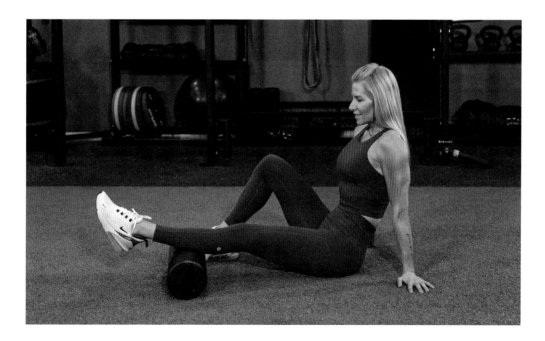

Hamstrings and Adductors

Benefits

The hamstrings help to extend the hip while controlling motion at the knee and adductors, which work to flex and extend the hip. When the hamstrings become too tight, they can change the position of the pelvis and ultimately affect mobility of the hip joints. Myofascial release with a foam roller helps to reduce tightness, ensuring optimal mobility and function of the hips.

Instructions

1. Sit with your legs directly in front of you and your hands under your shoulders. Keep your spine long and straight.
2. Place the back of your left thigh on top of the foam roller and slowly move your leg forward and backward to find a tight or tender spot (this is where bundles of muscle fibers have become tight; you'll know it when you feel it).
3. Once you find a tender spot, roll on it for 15 to 20 seconds while rotating your leg to point your foot toward and away from the midline of your body before moving on to find another tender spot. Repeat for a total of 45 to 60 seconds before switching legs. Spend the same amount of time on both legs.

Correct Your Form

When your left leg is on the foam roller, bend your right leg to place your right foot flat on the ground and use your leg to help support your body weight. If holding yourself off the ground causes too much soreness on the back of the leg or your wrists, you can remain seated on the ground. It is not uncommon for the muscles of one leg to feel tighter than the other, but make sure to spend the same amount of time on both legs.

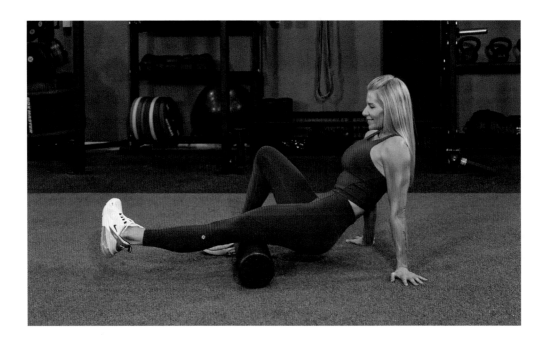

Quadriceps and Hip Flexors

Benefits

When the quadriceps or hip flexors become too tight, they could create an anterior (forward) tilt of the pelvis and alter the function of the hip joints. Using myofascial release to reduce tightness in the large quadriceps muscles can ensure optimal motion of the hip and function of the knee.

Instructions

1. Lie face-down, supporting your weight on your elbows. Straightening your legs behind you, place the front of your left thigh on the roller; move forward and backward until you locate a tender spot.

2. Continue rolling on the tender spot for approximately 15 to 20 seconds before moving to the next tender spot. Repeat for a total of 45 to 60 seconds, then switch legs. Spend the same amount of time on both legs.

Correct Your Form

Keep your elbows aligned directly below your shoulders and press them into the floor for stability. If your shoulders start to fatigue, you can lie down to perform the movement. Keep your spine long and extended. Try not to let your shoulders round or your chest collapse—that could place additional stress on your upper body.

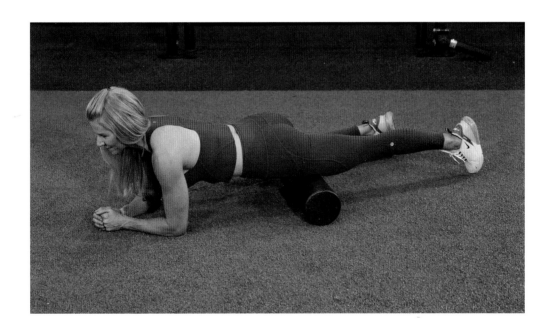

Lateral Quadriceps and Iliotibial Band

Benefits

The vastus lateralis is the most lateral of the four quadriceps muscles, and the iliotibial band is fascia that connects your pelvis to the tibia of the lower leg. When these tissues become tight, they could pull the knee out of alignment and affect how it functions in relation to the hip. Foam rolling these tissues helps to support optimal biomechanics of the lower body.

Instructions

1. Lie on your left side with your left elbow directly under your left shoulder. Start with the foam roller under the thigh, just above the knee.
2. Support your body weight with your elbow and by crossing the right leg over the left to place your right foot on the floor.
3. Slowly roll up and down the outside of the thigh. When you find a tight spot, roll on it for 5 to 10 seconds to help reduce the tightness. Repeat for a total of 45 to 60 seconds, then switch legs. Spend the same amount of time on both legs.

Correct Your Form

To reduce the pressure on the muscles of the left thigh, support more of your body weight with the right leg by pressing your right foot into the floor. To reduce tightness by increasing the pressure, place both legs on top of one another and support your body weight with only your elbow.

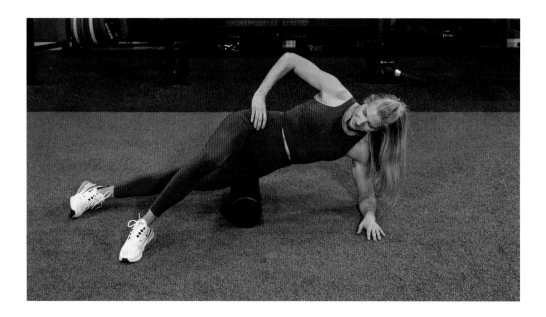

Latissimus Dorsi

Benefits

The large latissimus dorsi muscle of the back connects the pelvis to the arms and shoulders. The superior attachments on the humeral bones of the upper arms can create internal rotation at the glenohumeral joint of the shoulders; when this muscle is too tight, it can pull your shoulders forward, which could cause back pain. The inferior attachments at the posterior, superior portion of the pelvis can pull the pelvis up to create an anterior tilt and change mobility of the hip joints. Reducing tightness in the latissimus dorsi could help restore and maintain optimal mobility at both the shoulders and hips.

Instructions

1. Lie on your left side with your left arm lengthened and the foam roller close to your left armpit.
2. Slowly roll in the direction of your left hand. When you find a tight spot, slowly roll on it toward the front of your body, then lean back, bringing your left shoulder closer to the ground for 15 to 20 seconds. This creates cross-friction, which could help eliminate the adhesion. Then move to another tender spot on the muscle.
3. Repeat for a total of 45 to 60 seconds before switching sides of the body. Spend the same amount of time on both sides.

Correct Your Form

Keep your arm extended straight overhead to ensure the ability to find a tight or tender spot. Use your right hand to help support your body weight.

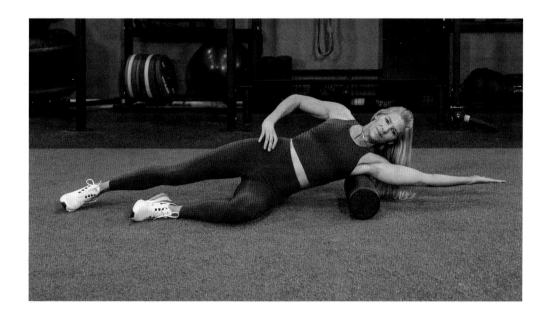

Lower and Middle Back

Benefits

When the muscles and connective tissues of the lower back become overly tight, they can change the position of the pelvis and limit mobility of the hip joints. Reducing tightness in these muscles can help to ensure optimal motion of both the upper back and the hips. Besides being a great recovery move for lower back muscles, this is also an excellent way to reduce tightness as part of a warm-up after being seated all day.

Instructions

1. Place the roller under your middle back. Place your feet flat on the floor with your knees pointed toward the ceiling to help support your body weight.

2. Slowly roll toward and away from your feet. When you find a tender or tight spot, roll on it for 15 to 20 seconds while slowly flexing and extending your spine before moving to find another tight spot. Repeat for a total of 45 to 60 seconds.

Correct Your Form

Place your tailbone on the ground if you are having too much trouble supporting your body weight with your legs. Move your feet away from your tailbone if the hamstring muscles along the backs of your legs start cramping.

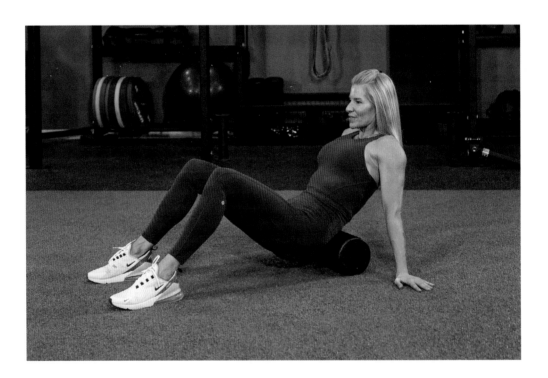

Recovery From the Inside Out

Accumulated stresses from repetitive exercises, exercises performed with poor technique, or a lack of multiplanar movement in general affects your body on many different levels and could keep you from achieving optimal performance. On the cellular level, force regulation can change the physical properties and biochemical function of muscle cells (Ingber 2004; Schleip et al. 2012; Vogel and Sheetz 2006). The mechanical forces imposed on your body during high-intensity exercise can change how the components of your myofascial system function on both the macro and micro scales, which explains why proper tissue-treatment strategies for recovery are so critical. Structure dictates function; if forces such as compression, tension, torsion, or shear enter the system and are not properly balanced, they could change the architecture of cellular structures, which ultimately changes the overall function of your body. The myofascial network is designed to be moved in all directions at a variety of different velocities; nutrition, hydration, and lifestyle habits such as proper sleep all affect the hydration and elasticity of muscle and connective tissues. A lack of multiplanar movement and proper hydration can cause layers of fascia to bind, creating adhesions and changing the body's ability to move efficiently. Making foam rolling a consistent part of your workout program can help to ensure optimal recovery between hard workouts.

Exercise is a function of movement, and movement is a function of numerous muscles working together to propel joints through their structural range of motion. If you are training for an activity that requires repetitive, linear movements, a low-intensity workout of multidirectional mobility exercises the day after a hard workout could help to ensure optimal resilience and function of your connective tissues. A low-intensity, multiplanar recovery workout is especially important if you are a bodybuilder or figure competitor, because exercise programs based on isolated body parts do not engage the elastic ability of the fascia to move in multiple directions. The day after a hard workout, multidirectional movements at a slow tempo could ensure optimal hydration and circulation of blood through the tissues to facilitate the repair process in all layers of the myofascial network.

PART II

STRATEGIES FOR OPTIMAL RECOVERY

6

IMMEDIATE RECOVERY: THE FIRST 24 HOURS

How many times have you caught yourself mindlessly scrolling YouTube, Instagram, or TikTok videos on your phone? As a result of your binge, the battery drops to low levels and requires a recharge. Streaming too many videos will rapidly drain the battery on your phone, and you will need to either allow time for the phone to recharge or carry an additional battery pack so you do not run out of charge. Think of high-intensity exercise as like watching videos on your phone; it can quickly deplete your muscles' available energy.

High-Intensity Exercise Drains Your Battery

Just like your phone battery after hours of watching videos, completing a high-intensity workout means your muscles are drained of energy and will need time to completely recharge. The good news is that you can take certain steps to accelerate the recharging process so you can begin your next hard workout or competition completely recovered, with a "full battery" of energy in your muscles (meaning you have allowed enough time for complete restoration of glycogen stores in muscle cells).

Recharging Your Battery

Whew. The workout is done. Over. Finished. It was a tough one, and you pushed yourself to complete every single repetition. Now you're feeling drained and mentally exhausted. The truth is that you like this feeling. This is why you exercise. However, now that the workout is over, what do you do next? If it's the morning, do you just head off to work and go on with your day? If you worked out in the evening, do you just go home and start getting ready for bed? Do you have a healthy snack or protein drink ready and available? Do you wear any special compression clothing or do any specific tissue treatment to promote recovery? Yes, you just did a tremendous amount of exercise in pursuit of your goal; however, now that the workout is over, it's time to get ready for the next one with specific strategies that will help you recover and prepare you for the next challenging training session. What you do immediately after one workout can promote a rapid return to homeostasis so that you can be 100 percent recovered and ready to go before your next workout or competition.

How High-Intensity Exercise Causes Muscle Damage

Even if you are a professional athlete during a competitive season who does a skills practice in the morning and a conditioning session in the afternoon and competes most weeks during a multimonth season, it is very unlikely that you are exercising more than 4 or 5 hours a day, 6 days a week, which would total up to 30 hours of exercise. There are 168 hours in a week, which means that even if you are training at the upper limits of human performance, you spend more time in postexercise recovery than actually exercising.

According to common gym mythology, strength training works by damaging muscle fibers, which are then repaired to become larger and capable of generating greater amounts of force. This is essentially true, but like many things with the human body, what actually happens is much more nuanced and complicated. High-intensity exercise does indeed cause muscle damage; muscle fibers slide against one another to produce contractions, causing damage to the mechanical structures of the fibers, which in turn signal satellite cells, proteins, and anabolic hormones to initiate the repair process. In addition, metabolizing the energy to fuel high-intensity muscle contractions results in individual muscle cells depleting stored glycogen; the by-products of anaerobic metabolism, which include lactate, hydrogen ions, and creatine kinase, can accumulate to create the sensation of fatigue and disrupt a muscle's ability to generate force. That burning sensation you may feel in your muscles during intense exercise indicates an accumulation of metabolic by-products that change blood acidity, and it is the first sign of the onset of fatigue. In addition to indicating that a muscle has exhausted its supply of energy, fatigue is a sign of reduced levels of electrolytes such as calcium, sodium, and magnesium, which play an important role in facilitating muscle contractions. The loss of energy substrates and electrolytes combined with an accumulation of by-products from anaerobic metabolism can greatly reduce a muscle's ability to generate force.

Creating Balance Between Exercise and Recovery

One way to understand the need for recovery is to apply the third law of physics, which states that for every action, there is an equal and opposite reaction. When high-intensity exercise is the action, the reaction is systemic overload and a complete disruption of homeostasis in the involved muscles and physiological systems. Once exercise is over, it is necessary to allow enough time for a complete return to a normal state of rest. No matter what your personal fitness goals are, achieving *any* goal with exercise requires finding an appropriate balance between imposing the progressive overload that causes the desired adaptations and allowing the time to return to homeostasis, a sign that your body has completely recovered from the workout.

It can be easy to finish a workout and simply go on about your day, but when you perform moderate- to high-intensity exercise that could be rated as a level of 7 to 10 out of 10 on the rating of perceived exertion (RPE) scale and you feel fatigued or exhausted, your muscles have experienced both metabolic and mechanical stress, creating a significant disruption to homeostasis. For you to achieve the results you want from your workouts, once the exercise portion of a workout is over, it is time to start the recovery phase by applying specific strategies to promote the return to homeostasis by lowering body temperature, rehydrating, and replacing the energy expended during the workout.

As you determine the most effective recovery strategies for your particular needs, take ownership of this simple concept: The end of one workout is the start of the next.

After exercise is over, muscles are still consuming oxygen as they expend energy to remove metabolic by-products and begin the repair process. Excess postexercise oxygen consumption (EPOC) is the use of oxygen to restore the body to homeostasis and normal pre-exercise (resting) levels of metabolic function. It is an indication that your muscles are still active even though you have finished exercising. When exercise begins, initial energy needs are delivered via anaerobic pathways until a steady state of oxygen consumption is achieved and the aerobic energy system is able to provide most of the required energy. An oxygen deficit is the difference between the volume of oxygen consumed during exercise and the amount that would be consumed if energy demands were met only through the aerobic energy pathway. If the adenosine triphosphate (ATP) that is needed to exercise at a particular intensity is not obtained aerobically, then it must come from anaerobic pathways. When you turn your car off after a long trip, the engine takes a few hours to completely cool down, but your muscles are different because they are consuming oxygen during the cooling process; they are still burning calories while returning to homeostasis, whereas your car's engine is not using any more gasoline.

Excess postexercise oxygen consumption is influenced by the intensity of exercise, not the duration; during EPOC, muscles use an elevated amount of oxygen and burn additional energy to perform the following functions (LaForgia, Withers, and Gore 2006):

- Metabolize free fatty acids into ATP via aerobic metabolism (mitochondrial respiration)
- Metabolize glycogen from lactate
- Restore oxygen in the blood and skeletal muscle
- Repair damaged tissue (muscle protein resynthesis)
- Restore body temperature to the normal resting level

Coach the Workout Instead of Doing the Workout

An unfortunate side effect of working in the fitness industry is the risk of overtraining syndrome, which can lead to burnout and job dissatisfaction. If you work as a group fitness instructor or coach responsible for leading group workouts, you have to plan and lead large groups through their workouts but still need to complete your own, personal exercise. All of that exercise could easily result in overtraining syndrome; it can be very easy to get caught up in the energy and do the entire class yourself while you're leading it, but you have to remember, it's *their* workout, not yours.

Of course, it's exciting to lead workouts that help others improve their lives, but physically participating in every class you teach—especially high-intensity interval training formats—can be extremely demanding on your body and could easily result in overtraining syndrome, especially if you are not applying any specific recovery strategies immediately after you teach a class or complete your own workout. Think of yourself as a professional athlete; you need to maintain your body at an optimal level of performance so you can use it to generate an income. This means learning how to lead and coach workouts instead of doing them. Doing the workout with the class could help motivate the participants, but you still need to take care of yourself, which means learning how to coach classes without doing the workouts. The best strategy is to stop doing the classes and stay focused on coaching clients through the workout.

The use of timers makes this type of coaching very easy; simply demonstrate the exercise, then start the timer and observe students to ensure they are maintaining optimal form. If necessary, you can do a few repetitions with the group to get them through a tough part of the workout, but for the most part, they should be doing the exercise, not you.

When was the last time you ate out at a nice restaurant and the chef came and joined you at your table? It likely has not happened because the job of a chef is to prepare the meal, not eat it for you. Being an instructor is similar; your job is to prepare a workout and coach students through it, not perform the workout for them. Once you learn how to do that, your job satisfaction will increase, and the chances of developing overtraining syndrome will go down dramatically.

Accelerating the Return to Homeostasis

After high-intensity exercise, any method used to enhance the recovery process should emphasize elevating the heart rate and blood circulation for the purpose of delivering oxygen, nutrients, satellite cells, and tissue-repairing hormones to muscles while removing by-products like creatine kinase (an enzyme produced in response to muscle protein damage) or inflammatory agents like interleukin that could impair the tissue-repair and energy-replenishment processes (Dupuy et al. 2018; Hausswirth and Mujika 2013).

Immediately after a high-intensity workout, your focus should shift into repair and recovery mode. No matter how strenuous or intense your workout, implementing recovery strategies once you are finished can help accelerate the return to homeostasis and reduce the risk of becoming overtrained. Four general strategies can help mitigate acute inflammation and promote postexercise recovery by facilitating a rapid return to homeostasis: rehydrating, refueling, repairing (as in tissue repair), and resting.

Hydration

From lubricating joints to transporting nutrients via the bloodstream, water supports many vital functions in the human body. In addition, water is essential for helping reduce the heat generated by muscle contractions. These are among the many reasons why maintaining proper hydration is essential for achieving optimal physical performance. Proper hydration supports the blood volume necessary to move nutrients and oxygen to working muscles, helps to dissipate the heat generated by muscle contractions, and supports a rapid recovery from exercise. Excessive sweating during activity could result in a loss of calcium, sodium, potassium, and other electrolytes that play an important role in muscle contractions. Exercise-related cramping is often associated with low electrolyte and hydration levels, which means that low hydration, referred to as hypohydration, will affect performance during activity and increase the time to achieve a full recovery.

To help control the internal body temperature during exercise, the sympathetic nervous system (SNS) causes blood vessels near the surface of the skin to dilate, allowing heat and water to escape. During exercise, the average adult can sweat up to 1.5 liters (50 fl oz) of fluid per hour, and athletes can sweat up to 2.5 liters (85 fl oz) per hour when competing. The temperature, the environment, and an individual's sweat rate will influence the amount of water lost during activity. Water composes approximately 70 percent of muscle tissue and blood and is distributed within cells (intracellular fluid), between cells (interstitial fluid), and in plasma (intravascular fluid). When the body is at rest, approximately 40 percent of its total mass is intracellular fluid, 15 percent is interstitial fluid, and 5 percent is intravascular fluid (McDermott et al. 2017). Maintaining proper hydration levels allows your body to properly thermoregulate and remove the excess heat produced by exercise. Losing up to two percent of your body weight through sweat can result in a loss of performance; a four-percent loss of body weight from sweating will have a negative effect on your body's ability to perform normal physiological functions; and a loss of eight percent is an indication of severe heat stress and possible heat stroke. Hypohydration is a loss of body water as the result of dehydration; in athletes, losing two percent or more of their body weight during exercise could significantly impair performance and increase the length of time to return to homeostasis after exercise (Haff and Triplett 2016).

Hyperhydration

Proper hydration is essential for optimal physical performance; however, excessive hydration is unnecessary and, in fact, could even be fatal. Hyperhydration is a condition of excessive total-body water content that results in expanded intracellular volumes. Exercise-associated hyponatremia is recognized as serum sodium concentrations of less than 135 mmol/L during or within 24 hours of physical activity (McDermott et al. 2017). Exercise-associated hyponatremia occurs when there is too much water and not enough sodium to facilitate the water being absorbed into tissues. The result is that organs such as the brain could drown in the excessive liquid. Hydration is important, but unless it is hotter than normal or you will be exercising for more than an hour, it is not necessary to consume an excessive amount of water prior to exercise; following the guidelines established by the National Athletic Trainers' Association should provide you with the hydration to perform your best during activity and recover quickly afterward.

Water plays a critical role in the postexercise recovery process. The more quickly you can rehydrate, the more you will be supporting your body's return to homeostasis. Once you have completed a high-intensity workout or competition, it is necessary to replace water as soon as possible so you can start preparing for the next. In muscle cells, glycogen holds on to water; as glycogen is metabolized into ATP, it releases the water, which is then used to help control thermoregulation during exercise via sweat. In addition to significantly reducing a muscle's ability to contract and generate force, losing an excessive amount of water during exercise could put you at risk for heat stroke, which not only could affect your ability to exercise for a number of days but, depending on the severity, could actually be fatal.

Heat stress does not only occur in a hot environment. It can also happen when performing high-intensity physical activity in the cold. As muscles work in the cold, they still generate heat, and the body still gives off sweat. Not properly hydrating in a cold environment could result in heat stress because the body does not have enough water to maintain proper thermoregulation.

Your individual sweat rate will play a role in how you should hydrate during and after activity; the easiest method for monitoring your hydration status, besides the feeling of thirst, is to pay attention to the color of your urine. Urine color provides an indication of hydration levels; urine that is relatively clear, or light yellow, indicates proper hydration status, whereas darker urine usually indicates hypohydration. It is important to stay properly hydrated between workouts, and keeping track of the color of your urine is highly recommended when you will be doing more outdoor activity during the warmer months. For more information on how to monitor your hydration status, go to www.hydrationcheck.com.

Signs of Hypohydration

Early signs of exercise-related dehydration include a sensation of thirst combined with feelings of general discomfort or fatigue. One reason for exercise is to achieve and maintain a healthy body weight, and weight loss may be a goal worth striving for. However, significant weight loss should not occur during a single exercise session. Losing as little as two percent of one's body mass during exercise is an indication of hypohydration and potential heat stroke. Additional signs include the following (McDermott et al. 2017):

- Thirst
- Flushed skin
- Excessive sweating
- Dry mouth
- Fatigue
- Headache
- Muscle cramping

Replacing fluid immediately after exercise can help restore overall blood volume to pre-exercise levels, which in turn can reduce the time it takes to return to homeostasis.

Note that sport drinks containing glucose should only be consumed once you have started sweating. Consuming a drink high in sugar prior to exercise can elevate insulin levels, which will influence energy availability during exercise. It is best to wait until your body temperature is elevated and you have started sweating before consuming a sport drink or glucose-based gel. When your workout is going to last 45 to 50 minutes or less, water is all you need; however, if your workout is going to be longer than an hour, a glucose-based sport drink can be a valuable source of immediate energy to keep you moving.

Hydration for Immediate Recovery

The general strategy of hydration is to replace the water lost during exercise. In muscle cells, glycogen molecules attach to water; when glycogen is used to produce ATP, it releases the water, which becomes sweat that releases heat generated by muscle contractions. The first two hours after exercise is an important time frame for replacing the fluid, electrolytes, carbohydrates, and protein lost during activity; this can be done with a combination of hydration and nutrition.

Before Exercise
Drink up to 20 fluid ounces (0.6 L) of water in the two to three hours before starting your workout.

During Exercise
Drink 7 to 10 fluid ounces (0.2 to 0.3 L) of water every 10 to 20 minutes while exercising. During exercise, it is recommended to drink before feeling thirsty, so do your best to consume as much liquid as comfortably possible, especially when you are sweating.

After Exercise
When time allows, weigh yourself (after emptying your bladder) immediately before exercise and immediately after; then consume 1.5 liters of fluid (50 fl oz) for every kilogram of weight lost (or 0.7 liters [24 fl oz] for every pound of weight lost) (Haff and Triplett 2016).

During Exercise Lasting Longer Than 90 Minutes
If you exercise for an extended period of time, consuming a sport drink that contains branched-chain amino acids, in addition to glucose and electrolytes, could help reduce the risk of gluconeogenesis (the process of using protein to metabolize ATP), allowing more protein to be available to repair tissues once the workout is over.

There has been some recent debate about the need for excessive hydration during exercise. The bottom line is that muscle tissue and blood contain water. If hydration levels fall too low, it will affect performance. Postworkout recovery drinks not only can help rehydrate muscles but could also be an important source of macronutrients such as carbohydrates and proteins to help facilitate faster recovery. Protein drinks can be an effective means of delivering the protein that is essential for promoting muscle repair and, ultimately, growth. Table 6.1 provides more information about common recovery drinks.

TABLE 6.1   Common Beverages for Hydration Recovery

BEVERAGE	DESCRIPTION
Glucose- and electrolyte-based sport drinks	Electrolytes such as sodium, magnesium, and calcium help increase the permeability of muscle cell membranes, which makes it easier for water to enter the cells to ensure optimal hydration. Electrolytes also help with conduction of electricity from the nervous system to motor units that stimulates muscles to contract. A loss of electrolytes could impede optimal muscle function during exercise. During prolonged physical activity, especially during hot weather, because electrolytes facilitate the absorption of water, it is recommended to consume sport drinks that contain • 460-690 mg (0.02 oz) of sodium per liter, • 78-195 mg (0.003-0.007 oz) of potassium per liter, and • a carbohydrate concentration of 5%-10%. The muscles and liver contain only a finite amount of glycogen, which must be converted to glucose before being metabolized into ATP. If muscle cells run out of glycogen for ATP and glucose is not immediately available through the bloodstream, then cortisol is used to convert protein into ATP via a process called gluconeogenesis. High-intensity exercise that lasts longer than 45 or 50 minutes can deplete glycogen levels. Sport drinks containing glucose supply much-needed energy to maintain muscle contractions. By providing an immediate source of glucose that can be delivered to muscle cells, glucose-based sport drinks can help accelerate recovery immediately after high-intensity exercise, which is important from one practice or training session to the next or during a multigame tournament. The downside to glucose-based sport drinks is that they are high in calories. If you are exercising for weight loss, rehydrating by adding an appropriate amount of sodium to water may be the best option.
Pickle juice, cherry juice, and beet juice	Losing sodium from sweat can affect the ability of muscles to contract and could result in fatigue or cramps. Sport drinks add sodium, which can help muscle cells absorb water more effectively, but they also contain calorie-rich glucose. Some athletes drink the liquid found in jars containing pickles, cherries, or beets. The idea is that the high sodium in these liquids can promote recovery by increasing the speed of rehydration. It is interesting to consider who first discovered the concept of drinking pickle juice. You'd have to be pretty thirsty to think that downing the brine from a jar of pickles would be a good idea. However, the belief is that drinking pickle or beet juice could be an effective means of recovery because it contains high levels of sodium, an electrolyte that helps water pass through the membranes of muscle cells more easily and is important for rehydration. Drinking pickle or beet juice is a relatively new approach to recovery, so the evidence is limited. MacKenney and colleagues (2015, 141-146) saw no significant changes in plasma sodium up to 120 minutes after drinking pickle juice. Likewise, Miller, Mack, and Knight (2009, 454-461) found that ingesting pickle juice did not cause significant changes to electrolyte concentrations in the blood. Nevertheless, if you don't mind the taste, this could be an effective recovery approach on very hot days when you lose a lot of fluid through sweat.
Protein drinks, recovery shakes, and chocolate milk	Consuming a drink containing both protein and carbohydrate immediately after high-intensity exercise could help to accelerate the muscle repair and recovery process. According to a review of the research, the addition of protein to a carbohydrate-based recovery drink could reduce the amount of muscle damage and delayed-onset muscle soreness (Pritchett, Pritchett, and Bishop 2012). The carbohydrates in a recovery drink can elevate insulin levels to ensure that glucose is properly stored in muscle cells (as glycogen), whereas the protein can provide important macronutrients for repairing tissues damaged during exercise. If a protein drink or recovery shake is not available, chocolate milk could be an effective solution. Research suggests that chocolate milk contains an effective ratio of protein to carbohydrates that could help support postexercise recovery (Lunn et al. 2012).

Abbreviation: ATP, adenosine triphosphate.

Nutrition

In relation to the postexercise recovery process, *when* nutrition is consumed in relation to exercise may be more important than *what* is consumed. After moderate- to high-intensity exercise, a snack, shake, or meal supplement containing healthy sources of carbohydrates and protein could help promote the recovery process by replenishing glycogen in the muscle cells while facilitating the repair of tissues damaged during exercise. Consuming a postexercise snack, meal, or drink with the recommended carbohydrate-to-protein ratio and within the suggested time frame could help you recover from the day's workout and prepare your muscles for tomorrow's activity.

When you know you are going to be doing high-intensity exercise, it is a good idea to plan for how you will fuel within the first hour or so after finishing the workout. High-intensity exercise drains the energy from your muscles; the immediate focus of postworkout nutrition should be replacing that energy. When it comes to nutrition for recovery, the purpose is to supply enough nutrients for optimal energy and tissue repair; if you require a specific diet, it is a good idea to work with a registered dietitian-nutritionist, who can help you develop a meal plan for your specific needs.

Nutrition for recovery should deliver enough protein and carbohydrates to muscles for them to quickly repair and refuel in order to be ready to function at a high level of performance. Training to achieve optimal performance is not the time to cut calories. If you do need to cut calories to make a specific weight, it is best to work with a sports dietitian, who can provide the proper guidance. When it comes to recovery, the purpose of nutrition is to refuel muscle cells, promote the repair of damaged muscle tissues, and support a healthy endocrine system, which produces the hormones responsible for repairing muscle proteins. High-intensity workout programs are popular because they are an effective and efficient way to burn a lot of calories while sculpting well-defined muscles. However, doing too much high-intensity exercise too frequently without proper recovery nutrition could increase the risk of developing overtraining syndrome. Exercise drains the gas from your tank; proper recovery nutrition provides the high-octane fuel that allows you to perform your best.

Food Is Energy

A calorie is the amount of energy required to increase the temperature of one liter (34 oz) of water by one degree centigrade. The calorie count of food indicates how much energy it provides. The first law of thermodynamics states that energy is neither created nor destroyed; it is merely transferred from one form to another. Energy consumed in the diet will either be used immediately to support your body's metabolic functions or stored as fatty acids in adipose tissue to be used later. Whether you are running or cycling for long distances, lifting really heavy stuff, or playing a team sport, nutrition provides the energy for you to move. High-intensity exercise is fueled by anaerobic metabolism, which depletes the amount of carbohydrate (stored as glycogen in muscle cells) available for other activities. Breathing rapidly and sweating during exercise indicate that glycogen is indeed being metabolized for energy. Your breathing rate increases to remove carbon dioxide; glycogen attaches to water in muscle cells, and when it is metabolized into ATP, it releases the water, which turns into sweat. Consuming protein after exercise is essential for repairing the muscle tissue damaged during high-intensity contractions.

Your body's metabolism is responsible for converting the nutritional substrates from your diet into fuel for muscle contractions and for new cells that repair tissue damaged during exercise. During rest and low-intensity exercise, energy in the form of ATP is provided via free fatty acids through aerobic metabolism. However, the energy for high-intensity exercise is metabolized from anaerobic glycolysis, which places a significant demand on the involved muscle cells to rapidly produce the necessary ATP while depleting the amount of glycogen available. Regardless of whether it is resistance training or cardiovascular conditioning, one of the outcomes of high-intensity exercise is an extreme amount of stress caused by the metabolism of carbohydrates into ATP.

Nutrition Before and During Exercise

Recovery nutrition is not just what you eat after you exercise. Proper nutrition before and during a workout could also reduce your recovery time. Research indicates that consuming protein or branched-chain amino acids before and during high-intensity exercise could help promote the recovery process once exercise is complete. Ensure enough macronutrient intake to replace the energy expended during exercise (carbohydrates), support the process of muscle repair (protein), and help promote a healthy endocrine system (fat) (Kersick et al. 2017). According to a review of the literature by Pritchett, Pritchett, and Bishop (2012), the rate of muscle glycogen resynthesis is elevated during the first 6 hours after exercise, and it can take up to 24 hours to re-establish glycogen stores to normal resting levels.

Consuming All Macronutrients

For optimal energy levels and to support your overall exercise needs, the food consumed in your daily diet should provide adequate levels of protein, carbohydrates, and fat. Protein is used to repair damaged muscle fibers and produce new tissues, while the purpose of fat and carbohydrates is to provide energy for cellular activity, including that of muscle cells. A well-balanced diet requires appropriate levels of fat and carbohydrates to support vital physiological functions and provide energy so the body can achieve optimal performance.

The human body can store excess energy as fat in adipose tissue, but it can store only a limited amount of carbohydrates. This is why it is so essential to consume carbohydrates as part of the recovery process; muscles need to replace their energy stores. The liver can store between 75 and 100 grams (3 to 4 oz) of carbohydrates, which can produce up to 400 calories of energy (at 4 calories per gram). Approximately 300 to 500 grams (11 to 18 oz) of carbohydrates (1,200 to 2,000 calories) can be stored as glycogen in muscle cells (the amount of lean muscle tissue you have can influence the ability to store glycogen). Additionally, the bloodstream can contain 15 to 20 grams (0.5 to 0.7 oz) of circulating glucose (Arent et al. 2020). This is one reason why proper nutrition is so essential during the recovery process after high-intensity exercise; so much energy is expended that it is necessary to replace it as soon as possible so your muscles can be properly fueled and ready to function for the next high-intensity workout.

A healthy diet should not only focus on protein and carbohydrates but should contain adequate amounts of monounsaturated and polyunsaturated fats while limiting the amount of saturated and trans fats. Consuming excessive amounts of fats and carbohydrates, especially foods high in saturated or hydrogenated fats and sugar, is what leads to weight gain, not the macronutrients themselves. Don't think of fats or carbohydrates as things to avoid; instead, think of them as vital sources of energy for your body, essential for achieving optimal performance.

Nutrient Timing

The concept of nutrient timing refers to consuming nutrients in relation to your workout schedule so you have the optimal amount of fuel during your activity and your muscles can refuel once you're done. According to Arent and colleagues (2020), "Nutrient timing involves manipulation of nutrient consumption at specific times in and around exercise bouts in an effort to improve performance, recovery, and adaptation" (1).

Exercise increases the levels of hormones related to energy metabolism; consuming nutrition immediately after exercise can take advantage of these changing hormone levels in an attempt to promote a faster recovery. The period following exercise provides an ideal opportunity for timed nutrient intake to promote the restoration of muscle glycogen and protein synthesis while helping to reduce muscle protein breakdown. Postexercise nutrient timing may be an essential aspect of an optimal training program, because it has the potential to improve the rate of recovery and maximize training adaptations (Arent et al. 2020).

Kersick and colleagues (2017) summarized the state of research on nutrient timing in the International Society of Sports Nutrition's position stand on timing of nutrition:

> **Nutrient timing is an area of research that continues to gather interest . . . In reviewing the literature, two key considerations should be made. First, all findings surrounding nutrient timing require appropriate context because factors such as age, sex, fitness level, previous fueling status, dietary status, training volume, training intensity, program design, and time before the next training bout or competition can influence the extent to which timing may play a role in the adaptive response to exercise. Second, nearly all research within this topic requires further investigation . . . In its simplest form nutrient timing is a feeding strategy that in nearly all situations may be helpful towards the promotion of recovery and adaptations towards training (15).**

Chapter 9 will provide more information on nutrient timing strategies that can ensure you have a full tank of energy for your next workout or competition.

Tissue Repair

High-force, explosive, repeated muscle contractions damage muscle fibers and signal the immune system to initiate the repair process. Proper tissue treatment during the immediate postexercise recovery phase can help improve circulation to remove the by-products of anaerobic metabolism as well as reduce the buildup of collagen cells that could cause adhesions between layers of muscle tissue. Specific strategies can enhance circulation to remove metabolic by-products and markers of muscle damage from muscle tissue while delivering the oxygen, nutrients, immune cells, and hormones required for optimal tissue repair.

Your muscles and elastic connective tissues can experience a tremendous amount of mechanical stress during a high-intensity workout; postexercise tissue treatment can help improve circulation to remove the by-products of anaerobic metabolism and support the process of repairing tissues damaged during exercise. Various methods of tissue treatment can facilitate the return to homeostasis, promote tissue repair, and ensure an optimal recovery process. The general goals of tissue treatment are to reduce inflammation and increase circulation, bringing more oxygen and nutrients to working muscle tissue while removing the by-products of anaerobic metabolism (which could cause delayed-onset muscle soreness). Inflammation is a part of the normal recovery process and is essential for supporting tissue repair; however, chronic inflammation could overwork the immune system and leave it compromised and susceptible to outside invaders.

Foam Rolling

As explained in chapter 5, the natural inflammation that occurs during the tissue-repair process, combined with a lack of movement after an exercise session, could be a cause of muscle adhesions. Muscle damage from high-intensity exercise signals the repair process. This is when new collagen molecules are formed to help repair and strengthen tissue. If tissues remain in a relatively static, stationary position, then collagen could bind between the layers of muscle. Muscle damage can change the firing patterns of the motor units responsible for muscle contractions and the sequence in which muscles are recruited and engaged to produce a movement (MacDonald, Penney et al. 2013). Using a foam roller can help minimize the risk that the new collagen will form adhesions between muscle layers and can possibly increase the speed of postexercise recovery.

When using a foam roller, move at a consistent tempo of approximately one inch (2.54 cm) per second while remaining on areas of tension for up to 90 seconds to allow the tissue to relax and lengthen. Self-myofascial release using a foam roller can also elevate tissue temperature, which can help you prepare for a recovery workout the day after a hard training session.

Heating and Cooling Methods

Aside from foam rolling, table 6.2 lists other methods of helping tissue to recover.

There is a reason why many health clubs have saunas, steam rooms, and hot tubs: The heat from these relaxing environments helps promote postexercise recovery in muscles. Heat increases the body's circulation to remove metabolic by-products such as hydrogen ions and inorganic phosphates while carrying oxygen and other nutrients necessary to help repair tissue used during the workout. Another less comfortable but extremely effective option is the application of cold. Ice baths, ice packs, cooling vests, special chairs with pockets for ice packs,

TABLE 6.2 Additional Methods of Tissue Recovery

METHODS	HOW THEY WORK TO PROMOTE RECOVERY
Saunas, hot tubs, and steam rooms	Elevate body and tissue temperature to increase the heart rate
Cryotherapy and cold exposure	Increase circulation and reduce inflammation
Mechanical pressure	Increase circulation and reduce tightness
Compression clothing and pneumatic pressure sleeves	Help promote circulation via enhancing the return of deoxygenated blood from muscles back to the lungs to be reoxygenated
Cupping and scraping	Increase localized circulation and reduce inflammation
Static stretching	Reduce muscle tightness or soreness so joints have full range of motion

or cryofreeze chambers are all options for applying cold treatment. One benefit of cold treatment is that it can help reduce the body's core temperature. This is essential when exercising in hot weather or two or more times on the same day. A second benefit is that cold treatment can reduce inflammation and promote healing in tissue used during the workout.

Some of these methods are expensive, whereas other methods are more affordable and can easily be done at home while binge-watching your favorite television streaming service. Let's look at each option in more detail.

Heat Immersion

Heat immersion methods, such as infrared saunas, standard saunas, hot tubs, and steam rooms, increase the ambient temperature to elevate tissue temperature. As the tissue temperature rises, the heart rate will increase to help with thermoregulation; this increase in heart rate helps to promote recovery.

Unlike traditional saunas that use rocks or metal heating elements, infrared saunas heat with electromagnetic lamps (Hausswirth and Mujika 2013). An infrared sauna elevates tissue temperature, which can increase circulation to promote recovery. Infrared rays produce heat that molecules can partially absorb. Because the heat affects the cells directly, infrared saunas operate at a lower temperature, allowing for a more comfortable yet beneficial experience.

Cold Exposure and Cryotherapy

Ice baths promote recovery by increasing circulation, but some people do not want to spend 15 to 20 minutes in ice water to receive these benefits. An alternative is to visit a cryotherapy freeze chamber. Cryotherapy is the application of extremely cold temperatures (–110 to –140 degrees Celsius [–166 to –220 degrees Fahrenheit] for 2 to 4 minutes). There are two prevailing theories about how cryotherapy promotes recovery:

1. Exposure to extremely cold temperatures causes blood to rush to the vital organs to protect them. As the cold is removed and the body returns to normal temperature, the blood returns to the extremities, bringing necessary oxygen, nutrients, and cells. The rapid application of cold also causes the sympathetic nervous system to release epinephrine and cortisol, which increase circulation.

2. Cold helps reduce inflammation caused by mechanical damage to the tissue structures. Inflammation increases pressure on the nerve endings that sense pain; when inflammation is lowered, so is the perception of pain (Hausswirth and Mujika 2013).

Mechanical Pressure

Believe it or not, different mechanical-pressure modalities—percussion guns, self-myofascial release with foam rollers or hand-held sticks, and massage therapy—rely on the same basic idea: applying pressure to muscle tissue can increase circulation and reduce tightness. As mentioned in chapter 5, Golgi tendon organs (GTOs) are sensory nerve endings located where muscles attach to tendons. Have you ever been straining really hard to lift a weight, and then your muscles just gave out? That was the GTOs working to protect your muscles from damaging themselves. The GTOs respond to an increase in tension by causing muscle fibers to relax and lengthen—in essence, shutting a muscle down.

As chapter 5 explains, using a tool like a massage stick, foam roller, or percussion gun or working with a massage therapist is just another means of applying pressure to muscle tissue. This applied pressure initiates a reflexive response that lengthens muscle fibers, helping to reduce overall tightness. In the case of massage, the therapist can help increase circulation by working between the layers of tissue.

Percussion guns have become more affordable and easier to buy, making them a popular recovery tool; in fact, some health clubs invest in percussion guns and make them available for personal trainers working with clients or for members who pay an additional fee for access to a recovery room. The application of compressive force against muscle and connective tissues can provide a number of benefits, including increasing circulation, breaking up collagen fibers, reducing muscle tightness, and promoting localized blood flow to aid in tissue repair. The pressure from the gun can reduce neural drive in muscle fibers, allowing them to return to a normal resting length.

Compression Clothing

Wearing compression clothing before and after a tough workout is a relatively new strategy that may reduce the amount of time needed for optimal recovery. Compression clothing applies a steady source of pressure to muscle tissue that could help increase circulation by promoting venous return of blood to the heart. The pressure from the tight clothing can theoretically improve circulation, which helps remove metabolic by-products from muscle more quickly and promotes the flow of oxygenated blood to help tissue repair and rebuild. Compression clothing can also elevate tissue temperature, which could help reduce the overall perception of soreness (Dupuy et al. 2018).

Compression clothing also can help elevate tissue temperature, which in turn can reduce soreness. While there has been a variety of research on the effectiveness of compression clothing, there is no overwhelmingly conclusive evidence for or against it. One study observed no significant performance differences from wearing compression clothing (Duffield et al. 2008); however, a later study found that wearing compression clothing during and after exercise resulted in noticeable, albeit minor, changes in performance (Born, Sperlich, and Holmberg 2013).

Pneumatic Air-Pressure Cuffs

Pneumatic air pressure on the legs can increase overall circulation to promote venous return of blood to the heart. This can help remove metabolites while delivering fresh oxygen and nutrients to lower-body muscles.

Cupping and Scraping

Cupping is an ancient medicinal practice that places small glasses or bowls directly on the body to create suction on the skin and tissues underneath. Scraping uses special edged instruments to place pressure along fascial lines in an effort to stimulate the tissue-repair process. The pressure from both the cupping and the scraping methods increases localized circulation and produces an anti-inflammatory response, which promotes the healing that is essential to recovery (Weinberg 2016).

Static Stretching

Static stretching is the most basic form of tissue treatment. Holding a muscle in a lengthened position sends a signal to the GTOs that allows muscle fibers to lengthen. Static stretching by holding body parts in positions for 30 to 45 seconds at a time, either immediately after a workout or in the evening a few hours later, could help to reduce overall feelings of muscle tightness or soreness to ensure that joints can move completely through their intended ranges of motion.

Case Study: After-Workout Recovery

It is two months into the six-month race season, and Allison has been racing every other weekend and doing well, winning one 5K (3 mi) and finishing third in her first 10K (6 mi) of the season. Allison uses the following training schedule during a season; this is the first season where she is implementing specific recovery strategies after each training session.

Sunday

Race; if no race, an active rest day—a long walk or bike ride. On race days, once she is finished, Allison's recovery practice is to foam roll her leg muscles, spend time in an infrared sauna or a hot tub, eat a nutritious dinner, and then use a percussion gun on her muscles before hopping into bed an hour earlier than normal while wearing her compression pants.

Monday

Recovery run (1 to 2 miles [2 to 3 km] if she ran a 5K, 3 to 4 miles [5 to 6 km] if it was a 10K) and lower-body strength training. Allison performs lower-body mobility exercises before the strength training workout and uses a foam roller at the end of the workout to promote circulation and reduce tightness.

Tuesday

Interval training and upper-body strength training. Allison uses the percussion gun on her leg muscles and sleeps with her compression pants to help promote circulation.

Wednesday

Long run followed by two to three mobility exercises for the hips. Allison applies the percussion gun to her leg muscles and sleeps in her compression pants.

Thursday

Morning tempo run. At night, Allison does a yoga class to improve her mobility before using a foam roller or percussion gun and taking a cold bath, and she wears her compression pants to bed.

Friday

Short run and total-body strength training (circuit training). After the run and workout, Allison uses a foam roller on her legs to reduce overall muscle tightness.

Saturday

If racing on Sunday, rest and go to bed an hour earlier than normal. If no race, either a yoga class or a long hike followed by a trip to a massage therapist.

(continued)

After her workouts, Allison either uses her percussion gun or foam roller to reduce muscle tightness and promote circulation for optimal tissue treatment. In addition, Allison has been going to bed an hour earlier, especially the nights after her long runs and before her races, and she wears compression pants the night after a hard workout. Between the additional sleep and the use of compression pants, Allison notes in her training journal that she wakes up feeling completely recharged and ready to go. Finally, Allison has worked with her registered dietitian-nutritionist to identify the perfect preworkout and race snacks and the most effective recovery drink for immediately after a workout.

Allison credits her revamped nutrition immediately before and after her workouts, the use of the tissue treatment immediately after a workout, and the compression pants she wears while sleeping with giving her the ability to maintain a challenging yet effective training schedule, which has resulted in her reaching the podium in two of the four events she entered and finishing in the top 10 of her age group in the other two.

Sleep

Everyone who exercises on a regular basis wants the same thing: results. Consistent moderate- to high-intensity exercise is the most efficient means of causing desired changes to your body. However, what is often overlooked is that your approach to sleeping should be as mindful as your approach to exercise. One of the most effective methods for recovering from a hard workout is something you already do, but chances are that you may not do enough of it, or you may not use it to the fullest extent. A surefire method of promoting recovery so your exercise program produces the results you want is to get optimal sleep.

Your workouts can rock and leave you exhausted in puddles of sweat, and your nutrition can be dialed in, but if you don't get adequate sleep or practice effective sleep hygiene, then your workouts may not produce the desired results. Achieving results from any exercise program requires having a postworkout recovery strategy, and getting the optimal quality and quantity of sleep is one of the most efficient means of allowing your body to recover from a workout in order to be properly prepared for the next exercise session.

Allowing time for your body to achieve proper rest is not being lazy; it is a critical component of the recovery process. Your muscles do not get stronger or grow during a workout—it is after the workout that the growth and adaptations occur. Rest, specifically sleep, is when hormones such as testosterone and growth hormone are released to help support muscle protein synthesis and the repair process.

Proper sleep also strengthens the immune system. Sleep is when the body naturally detoxifies and repairs itself. An extra hour of sleep a night can result in an additional seven hours a week, which is like sleeping for an entire extra night. A lack of sleep can increase activation of the SNS and hypothalamus-pituitary-adrenal axis, which can suppress the immune system. "Sleep disturbances can depress immunity, increase inflammation, and promote adverse health outcomes," say Peake and colleagues (2017, 1084).

A full night's sleep allows time for anabolic hormones to perform the function of tissue repair, whereas insufficient sleep could result in higher levels of catabolic hormones responsible for energy production. If you have ever been completely exhausted but could not fall asleep, or if you do sleep but wake up not feeling completely rested, it could be the result of elevated SNS activity and higher levels of the hormone cortisol. The SNS governs your fight-or-flight response and releases cortisol, which helps convert free fatty acids into energy for exercise. However, when glycogen is in low supply, cortisol can also convert amino acids into ATP, which fuels muscle shortening and inhibits muscle growth.

One function of sleep is to allow time for muscles to repair themselves. Growth hormone is an anabolic hormone produced during stage three of non–rapid-eye-movement sleep and helps to repair tissues damaged during exercise; the longer a period of sleep, the more time for muscle tissues to regenerate and grow (Chennaoui et al. 2014).

Sleep is such a critical component of overall health that there is an organization of medical professionals and researchers who study and promote the benefits of sleep for achieving optimal health. This organization, the Sleep Foundation, recommends that adults get between seven and nine hours of sleep per night (Suni 2022). When it comes to planning your workouts, consider the end of one workout the beginning of the next. How you refuel, rehydrate, and sleep will allow you to be fully prepared so you can achieve the best results possible.

Sleep helps the body recover from metabolic overload, which occurs when muscles exercise to the point of fatigue, exhausting the amount of glycogen available for energy production. While you're sleeping, your body continues to digest carbohydrates from your diet and metabolize them into glycogen, which is then stored in muscle cells to fuel muscle contractions.

Another important benefit of sleep is that it allows time for the removal of unnecessary metabolic waste from brain cells. Being overly tired, especially during exercise, could result in reduced reflex times or poor judgment, each of which could cause a training injury. Think of sleep as the time when your brain is removing unwanted waste while enhancing blood flow to cells, bringing important oxygen and glycogen necessary for optimal cognitive performance.

Good sleep hygiene also promotes optimal function of the immune system. Outside of traumatic injury, illness can cause missed playing time for athletes, but you do not have to play sports to receive the benefit of avoiding illness. No matter what your job is, getting great sleep supports a strong immune system, which in turn reduces the risk of becoming sick, allowing you to optimize your performance and be more productive.

To ensure optimal performance during your workouts while putting yourself in the best position possible to reach your goals, it's a good idea to plan your workouts based on the sleep you'll be able to get each night. For example, if your evening plans include attending a concert, hitting a nightclub, or partying late into the night with friends, chances are that you will not achieve the recommended seven to nine hours of sleep. This does not mean you need to skip workouts, but it does mean scheduling your high-intensity workouts on days when you know you'll get great sleep and planning lower-intensity workouts on those days when you may have plans that will disrupt your normal nighttime routine and affect your ability to get adequate sleep. Taking your evening plans into account as you plan your workouts can help to ensure that you are properly prepared for the more challenging workout sessions that can provide the desired results.

If exercise is the period when stress is applied to the body, then consider sleep as the time when the body recovers from and adapts to the stresses imposed during the workout. This must be a harmonious relationship; too much exercise and too little sleep could result in overtraining, which at best could keep you from reaching your goals and at worst could lead to an injury that does not allow you to exercise at all.

Training goals will determine the overall training intensity and role of rest. If you're training for the Olympic qualifier and have one meet to qualify for a shot at Olympic gold, then you really need to watch your overall fatigue and recovery the closer you get to competition time. However, if you have general fitness goals and no specific time frame, you will want to make sure to schedule lower-intensity workouts during your week to keep your overall training load in check. Here's the good news for exercise enthusiasts: You *can* exercise every day. However, in order to be the most successful and reduce the risks of overuse or overtraining, it is important to alternate intensity on a workout-by-workout basis.

Identifying the Best Recovery Strategies for Your Needs

Commit to this mantra: Tomorrow's workout starts at the end of today's. As you plan for your hardest, highest-intensity workouts, you will want to plan for which recovery strategies you will use once the workout is over. Preparing a proper snack or shake, taking the time at the end of a workout to reduce muscle tightness, sitting in a sauna, or wearing compression clothing are all options that could help facilitate a speedy return to homeostasis the day of a hard workout. The only way to identify the best method for your particular needs is through trial and error. Keep in mind that recovery after a hard training session or single competition is different than recovery during a high-intensity training cycle or multigame tournament.

If it's important to you, use a fitness tracker with a heart-rate monitor to measure how long it takes your heart rate to completely return to a normal resting state (the true resting heart rate is measured first thing in the morning upon waking). Then, try various combinations of different recovery methods to find which work best for your budget and schedule.

Resting after a hard workout allows muscles to replace glycogen and ATP that fuel activity during exercise. Exercising too frequently without proper recovery may not give the body enough time to rest and replace energy burned in a workout. However, some workouts do not require a focus on recovery, particularly low- to moderate-intensity sessions that do not overstress body tissues or deplete glycogen stores.

As soon as you have finished one workout, it is important to start preparing for the next one. Especially if today's workout pushed you to a point of fatigue, you will need to take specific steps to help your body heal from and adapt to the physical work you just performed.

The day after a hard workout should find you still feeling the effects of the previous day. If you applied the right recovery strategies, then you may be sore, but it should not be excessive or keep you from any physical activity, especially exercise. In fact, as you will learn in the next chapter, low-intensity, steady-state exercise the day after a hard workout can be one of the most effective recovery strategies available. Low-intensity activities such as walking or cycling at a comfortable pace, gentle yoga, bodyweight exercises, or low-intensity circuit weight training are all solutions that can help promote recovery the day after a hard workout. More information on how to structure recovery workouts will be addressed in chapter 7.

7

THE DAY AFTER A WORKOUT: EXERCISES FOR ACTIVE RECOVERY

"I wake up in the mornin' and I raise my weary head . . ." is the opening lyric of Jon Bon Jovi's "Blaze of Glory" and is the perfect descriptor for the first few moments that your eyes are open the morning after a hard workout. You wake up and lie in bed for a few deep breaths, taking stock of your body and checking in on each part to see how it's feeling before you get up and start moving for the day. You had a hard training session yesterday, and even though you rehydrated, had your recovery meal, did your foam rolling, and slept in your compression clothing, you still feel a little sore, especially in your legs. A common question the day after a very hard workout is, "Am I going to be sore all day, or is there anything I can do to reduce that soreness?"

In short, the answers are no and yes, respectively.

First, to answer the question of whether you have to live with a day of soreness, you may indeed feel sore upon waking, but you can take actions to reduce that soreness. Second, is there anything you can do to reduce the soreness you feel after a hard day in the gym? The answer to that is a definitive yes! One of the best methods of recovery is to achieve and maintain a high level of fitness in the first place; the better your level of fitness, which can refer to overall aerobic efficiency (the ability to deliver oxygen to working muscles) and muscular strength, the quicker you should be able to recover after a hard workout.

An essential component of recovery is delivering oxygen to your muscles, and exercising regularly will do just that as the result of improved aerobic efficiency. Every exercise session causes a number of short-term responses that take place either during or immediately after a workout and ultimately result in the long-term adaptations you are working toward. For example, an immediate response to high-intensity exercise is localized muscle fatigue resulting from depleting the glycogen stored in muscle cells. However, during the course of a consistent high-intensity exercise program, your muscles will adapt to become more efficient at storing glycogen and using it for anaerobic metabolism during exercise. They will also become more efficient at cleaning up waste products once the workout is over. Repeated strength training and high-intensity metabolic conditioning sessions cause muscle cells to adapt by storing more glycogen for anaerobic metabolism, allowing you to maintain a higher work rate for a longer period before reaching fatigue. Consistent workouts and adherence to a long-term exercise program that properly alternates intensity are the first steps for improving the ability to recover from hard workouts. The other steps are taken the day of and the day after a workout to promote immediate, short-term recovery from hard exercise.

Why You Are Sore

First, it is important to distinguish between soreness and pain. Pain is a sharp, extremely uncomfortable sensation that signals something is not right in your body. If you feel pain, then any plan to exercise should be cancelled and your focus should shift to resting for the day to allow your body to heal. If pain persists for more than three or four days, it would be a good idea to schedule an appointment with your health care provider to ensure you do not have a serious injury.

Some soreness or discomfort, on the other hand, is simply a sign that your muscles performed more physical work than they are accustomed to doing; as explained in chapter 1, discomfort is caused by delayed-onset muscle soreness (DOMS), a combination of fatigue and mechanical damage to the muscle fibers. The day after a hard workout, your immune system is working to remove the inorganic phosphates and other detritus remaining from anaerobic metabolism. You could still be experiencing short-term inflammation that will be ongoing throughout the day as your body completely returns to homeostasis. As a result, the goal for today's workout is to do enough movement to reduce that discomfort and promote both tissue repair and energy replacement so you can be ready to work at your maximal effort for your next high-intensity exercise session.

Rest Is Not a Four-Letter Word

Muscles generate the force to move your body. The previous chapters explained how high-intensity exercise imposes a tremendous amount of metabolic stress on muscles and how that disrupts homeostasis. Chapter 5 described the properties of the different types of muscle tissue and the benefits of daily tissue treatment such as foam rolling. This chapter will review the mechanical forces imposed on muscle fibers and elastic connective tissues, with an emphasis on how you can help promote tissue repair the day after a hard workout. If you love to exercise and have specific fitness-related goals, you may consider *rest* a four-letter word (literally and figuratively), but rest doesn't mean simply sitting on the couch and mindlessly scrolling your favorite social media feed for hours on end; it can refer to active rest, which includes almost any form of lower-intensity exercise that elevates the heart rate above normal resting levels.

Soreness the day after a hard workout is an indication that you have not completely returned to homeostasis, and it is most likely caused by an accumulation of by-products of anaerobic metabolism triggering an inflammatory response from your immune system. The immune system's response to high-intensity exercise causes inflammation in the muscles used during a workout. This inflammation applies pressure to nociceptors, the nerve endings responsible for sensing pain—hence, the discomfort you experience. Elevating your heart rate with low- to moderate-intensity exercise the day after a high-intensity workout can be an effective tactic for increasing circulation to remove metabolic by-products and reduce this inflammation. Active rest, in the form of lower-intensity exercise, can function as a pain reliever while promoting regeneration and growth of the tissues used in exercise.

What If You *Like* the Feeling of Soreness the Day After a Workout?

There is nothing wrong with a little discomfort or mild soreness the day after a hard workout. In fact, if the purpose of your exercise program is to make specific changes to your body, then that *should* be a normal feeling. However, you do not want to be so sore that it affects your ability to move or do your normal exercise program. Excessive soreness the day after an intense exercise session or competition could tempt you to skip your next workout, and that is not how to get better. Given that it can take up to 72 hours to fully recover from high-intensity exercise, it is important to know how specific strategies can help facilitate the return to homeostasis and which ones are best for your particular needs. Postexercise recovery does not just mean resting after exercise. Although rest, especially sleep, is an important component of recovery, specific postexercise recovery strategies should focus on elevating circulation to remove metabolites and markers of muscle damage, replacing energy, and rehydrating. The specific exercises you perform for your workouts are only one component of athletic success. Another important component is recovery, and one effective way to promote recovery is more exercise—specifically, low-intensity activity that elevates the heart rate slightly above normal, delivering more oxygen, nutrients, and healing hormones to damaged muscle fibers while removing unnecessary metabolic by-products.

Specific recovery strategies are most crucial for competitions (especially multigame, multiday tournaments) and for workouts that last longer than an hour, specifically those done at a level of intensity where you are out of breath for most of the workout. Moreover, recovery strategies like nutrient timing can provide a quantifiable benefit, such as delivering a specific amount of carbohydrates to replace those used during exercise. In contrast, compression clothing or the use of a percussion gun to reduce muscle tightness may help you feel better without providing a specific, measurable result. Some nontraditional methods are so new that there is little peer-reviewed research about them. Often, they are popular because of an extensive variety of anecdotal support from people claiming to feel benefits. Whether you use traditional or alternative recovery tactics, you need to be improving circulation to help remove the waste from muscle tissue and bring new oxygen and nutrients to support building new tissue.

The Study of One

When it comes to understanding how the human body works, scientific observation leads to hypotheses and identifies trends based on quantifiable evidence. Although it is impossible to know exactly why you might be sore the day after a hard workout, this section will identify potential causes of that soreness and how they can be treated. Research studies select a series of variables to test, then apply those variables to a population to identify trends that can be used in future practice. It will take some trial and error to identify the best recovery methods for your specific needs, which explains why having a consistent method of recording your workout and recovery data is so important; it will allow you to identify trends and place the most emphasis on the methods that deliver the greatest results. As the previous chapter stated, immediately after a hard physical effort, consuming proper nutrition, rehydrating, applying appropriate tissue-care strategies, and getting great sleep can all help to minimize potential soreness while promoting the return to homeostasis. However, after high-intensity exercise, it is likely that you could feel sore, and if you do, consider it a sign that your immune system is working to repair your body. Therefore, any physical activity should be at a lower intensity to allow the healing process to occur.

An ironic reality about exercise is that even though you may be sore from a workout, more exercise—specifically, low-intensity exercise—could be one of the most effective methods for reducing soreness and helping to speed up the recovery process.

Reasons you could be sore the day after a hard workout include the following:

- *Damage to muscle fibers.* This could cause metabolic by-products to be trapped in muscle cells, creating DOMS.
- *Inadequate hydration.* This not only could reduce the ability of layers of muscle tissue to slide against one another but also could limit the amount of metabolic by-product that can be removed from muscle cells. A combination of the two factors could increase the perception of soreness.
- *Insufficient sleep.* Growth hormone and testosterone are anabolic hormones produced during the deep rapid-eye-movement cycles of sleep, and they can help repair damaged muscle tissue and promote the growth of new muscle fibers. In addition, sleep is when the brain cleans and repairs itself; a lack of sleep could impair both cognitive and physical performance.
- *Improper nutrition.* Muscle cells need energy to function. Proper nutrition provides the energy for muscles to repair themselves while also replacing the energy stores for the next high-intensity bout of exercise, when anaerobic glycolysis will be the primary source of energy.

Active Rest

Active rest is the process of elevating your heart rate to increase circulation so the blood can remove metabolic by-products while delivering fresh oxygen and replacing glycogen in muscle cells. This explains why, when your body is still returning to homeostasis, low- to moderate-intensity exercise that increases circulation can be considered a method of tissue treatment. Walking, cycling (either on a stationary bike or a real one), swimming or other aquatic exercise, mobility exercises, or bodyweight strength training are all examples of low-intensity exercise that can elevate tissue temperatures and increase circulation without placing a tremendous amount of additional stress on the body. This is beneficial for promoting a complete recovery the day after a hard workout. Yes, when you first start exercising, you might be sore for the first few minutes, but think of that soreness as an indication that your body is repairing itself. Believe it or not, this movement could help reduce soreness more quickly than not moving.

Stability–Mobility Relationships in the Body

When you hear the word *flexibility*, you probably think of holding a specific muscle in a lengthened position. Known as static stretching, this practice can help reduce tightness in a muscle by minimizing nervous-system activity and causing the muscle to lengthen. Foam rolling, described in chapter 5, is one method of reducing nervous-system activity to increase muscle length; static stretching is just a different approach. Static stretches require you to hold a stable position with minimal movement so the muscle can relax and lengthen. This technique is perfect immediately after you exercise, as you begin to cool down and transition to the recovery phase of your workout.

The term *flexibility* has often been used to describe the ability of muscles to lengthen in order to allow joint motion—specifically, the ability of a joint to move through its structural range of motion. The term *extensibility* describes the mechanical ability of muscle and connective tissue to lengthen and shorten as joint motion is occurring. As muscle, fascia, and elastic connective tissues lengthen and shorten, they control the movement of a limb or body segment through its structural range of motion. Therefore, mobility should be thought of as a combination of flexibility and extensibility: the ability of the involved tissues to lengthen and shorten while controlling unrestricted joint motion.

Muscles play an important role in creating and controlling mobility. By shortening to create tension on the fascia and elastic connective tissues, muscles generate the internal forces that control the movement of the skeletal system. Here is a scary thought: If your exercise programs do not include multidirectional movements, then your muscle, fascia, and elastic connective tissues could lose the ability to efficiently store and release mechanical energy. Mobility is an important component of athleticism because it helps to ensure that muscle, fascia, and connective tissues remain pliable and elastic to allow joints to articulate through their full range of motion. This explains why tissue treatment, which includes maintaining hydration to allow layers of muscle tissue to slide over one another without restrictions, is such an essential component of a recovery program.

The human skeletal system contains joint structures that either provide stability or allow mobility, which is why mobility exercises should be the foundation of an active recovery workout program. Repetitive stress, especially when combined with high-intensity exercise, could increase inflammation of tissues, which in turn could change how joints function. Multidirectional mobility exercises the day after a challenging high-intensity workout could help ensure the ability of the mobile joints to allow unrestricted motion. Mobility exercises should move the mobile ankle, hip, thoracic spine, and glenohumeral joints through their structural ranges of motion, whereas the relatively stable knee, lumbar spine, and scapulothoracic joints provide the foundation for that movement to occur (table 7.1).

TABLE 7.1 **Strategies for Joint Mobility**

JOINT	LOCATION	FUNCTION	MOBILITY STRATEGIES
Foot and ankle complex	The foot has numerous joints that help ensure proper motion. The transverse tarsal joint, located between the heel bone (calcaneus) and the bones of the midfoot, plays an important role in helping the foot transition from a stable lever to a mobile force dissipator. The ankle is composed of the distal tibiofibular joint (the far end of the two bones in the lower leg) and the talocrural joint (the talus bone between the far ends of the tibia and fibula).	The foot and ankle function together during the gait cycle of walking or running. The foot transitions from being mobile when it hits the ground to a stable structure once the heel raises off the ground. As the body passes over the foot, the transverse tarsal joint creates a stable lever for propulsion, which helps create force for the next phase of the gait cycle. The ankle is designed to be mobile and experiences its greatest amount of mobility when the foot is on the ground as the body passes over it during the midstance phase of the gait cycle.	Reduce tightness in the calf muscles. Move the foot in multiple directions during exercises such as lunges to allow it to maintain optimal mobility in the many joints. When possible, enhance dorsiflexion. Use a massage stick, foam roller, or percussion gun to relax and lengthen the muscle tissue so the ankle can move through its full range of motion without any restrictions.
Knee	The knee joint connects the lower end of the thigh bone (femur) and the upper portion of the tibia in the lower leg.	The knee is a relatively stable joint that helps control motion between the segments of the upper and lower leg.	Reduce tightness of calf muscles to allow for proper range of motion of the foot and ankle complex. Reduce tightness in the quadriceps and lateral hip muscles to allow optimal function between the hip and knee.
Hip	The hip joint is where the femur of the thigh connects with the pelvis.	The hip allows mobility in three planes of motion during the gait cycle of walking or running. A loss of motion in any of these planes can cause the joints above or below the hip to attempt to allow the motion.	Sitting for a long time could cause the hip flexors to become stuck in a shortened position, which will change the function of the gluteal muscles; reduce tightness in the hip flexors to help ensure optimal mobility and function of the hips and gluteal muscles. During high-intensity running and weightlifting, the gluteal muscles can generate a lot of force, which creates metabolic by-products; use a massage stick, foam roller, or percussion gun to help ensure optimal length of the hip flexors while flushing out by-products and speeding up recovery time.
Lumbar spine	These joints are intervertebral segments of the lumbar spine.	The lumbar spine creates a platform of stability between the mobile joints of the hips and the intervertebral segments of the upper spine.	The muscles that surround the lumbar spine can become tight from overuse; use a massage stick or foam roller or perform ground-based mobility exercises to reduce tightness, which then reduces soreness while promoting recovery.

JOINT	LOCATION	FUNCTION	MOBILITY STRATEGIES
Thoracic spine	These joints are intervertebral segments of the thoracic spine.	The thoracic spine allows mobility for rotation as the arms swing forward and backward during the gait cycle. The intervertebral segments of the cervical and thoracic spine, the neck, and the midback allow most of the motion for rotation of the spine, whereas the structures of the lumbar spine are designed to move primarily forward and backward.	If the muscles that surround and control the thoracic spine become too tight, they can restrict rotation of the upper back, which in turn could cause pain in the lower back. Use a foam roller or do mobility exercises to help reduce tightness and promote circulation to ensure an efficient return to homeostasis.
Scapulothoracic	The scapulothoracic joint is where the shoulder blade sits on the thoracic spine of the middle and upper back.	The scapulothoracic joint creates a stable platform for movement of the shoulder and arm.	If the chest muscles become too tight, they can pull the shoulder blades forward, which restricts shoulder mobility in addition to being a potential cause of back pain. The large latissimus dorsi muscle attaches to the upper arms, and when it is tight, it can cause internal rotation of the shoulders and restrict overall mobility. Use a percussion gun, stretch the chest and latissimus muscles, or do mobility exercises to help reduce tightness and allow for optimal, pain-free mobility.
Glenohumeral	Also called the shoulder joint, this is where the head of the humerus, relatively the shape of a ball, rests on the glenoid fossa of the scapula, which creates a socket or cup.	One of the most mobile joints in the body, the glenohumeral joint allows multidirectional movement of the arm.	

Mobility Exercises
for Active Recovery Workouts

Some workouts need to be done at a high intensity to stimulate the changes you want to make to your body; however, the idea that *all* workouts must leave you gasping for air is absolutely false. Rather than pushing yourself to the point of discomfort with every workout, learn how to use lower-intensity bodyweight workouts to help you recover from high-intensity exercise. Yes, it's the high-intensity exercise that stimulates adaptations in your muscles and physiological systems; however, lower-intensity workouts can be a part of the postexercise recovery process to help alleviate any discomfort the day after a very hard workout (Hausswirth and Mujika 2013). Low- to moderate-intensity mobility workouts can also help reduce muscle tightness and improve blood flow after a long day of limited movement, such as being stuck in meetings or traveling to a competition. Knowing how to use low-intensity workouts as a method of recovery allows you not only to be more active, which is most likely inherent in

Case Study: The Day After a Race

Road races tend to take place on Sundays, which means that during the season, Saturdays are rest days and Mondays become active recovery days. Once Allison finishes a race, she immediately uses a foam roller on her leg muscles and visits a hot tub and infrared sauna to accelerate the return to homeostasis. In addition, Allison makes sure to eat a proper refueling meal and gets to bed an hour earlier than normal for extra sleep.

Despite applying these techniques and wearing compression pants to bed the night after a race, during the season, Allison still tends to feel a bit sore when she wakes up on Mondays, so she has learned how to scale back her recovery workouts. If she ran a 5K (3 mi) race, then she does a slow two-mile (3 km) run to flush her legs; if she ran a 10K (6 mi), she does a three- to four-mile (5 to 6 km) recovery run. To start her recovery run, Allison does two or three mobility exercises followed by 5 to 10 minutes of brisk walking, gradually building to a slow jogging pace. After the run, Allison performs a bodyweight strength training circuit for her lower body, featuring three sets of hip hinges, multiplanar lunges, and split-leg squats (she does each exercise at a slow tempo for 40 seconds, with minimal rest between exercises and 45 to 60 seconds of rest after completing the entire circuit), followed by the use of a foam roller to reduce overall lower-body muscle tightness.

In previous seasons, Allison did not take an active recovery day and instead simply continued with her training intensity and volume on the day immediately after a race. Allison used to think that if she was tired, it was an indication that she needed to train harder. This season, however, Allison can tell the difference that the structured rest is making and is instead taking the approach that if she is feeling fatigued or if her workouts start slipping, she should adjust her training to lower the intensity as opposed to trying to work through the fatigue. Another benefit of her focused approach to recovery is that Allison gives herself permission to skip a workout if she is feeling tired or fatigued; rather than beat herself up for not doing the work, Allison recognizes that fatigue is an indication that she is not fully rested, so rather than try to push through and risk a training injury, she respects her body and gives it the rest it needs. The result is that she starts every race feeling strong and energetic with a full tank of gas, and her times are getting better with every race.

your DNA, but also to minimize overall stress on your body. Plus, for those who truly abhor a rest day, a low-intensity mobility workout can create the perception of being active and leave you feeling great until your next hard training session.

On the days when you feel tired or fatigued after a hard training session, you might be surprised by how a low-intensity bodyweight workout can recharge your batteries and boost your energy levels almost immediately. Even when you're tired and it feels like your legs each weigh a ton, once you start moving, you will most likely feel better and experience a burst of energy as the oxygen hits your muscles.

It is helpful to think of the stretch–shorten cycle as a rubber band; if stretched and held in a lengthened position before being released, the rubber band (or muscle) won't produce the same amount of explosive force as if it is rapidly pulled and immediately released. Combining tissue-treatment strategies with mobility training as a recovery strategy could ultimately help improve overall force production during exercise by reducing the transition time between lengthening and shortening, ultimately increasing muscle-force output (Verkoshansky and Siff 2009). Multiplanar movements at a variety of rhythmic speeds increase heat in the body, which helps layers of fascia and muscle to slide over one another, especially when they are well hydrated. Mobility exercises are a form of dynamic stretching that can help reduce muscle soreness and tightness, which could be a possible cause of injury. A recovery workout that includes low-intensity, multidirectional movement could also help to increase hydration of the tissues, which is essential for enhancing the elasticity and structural integrity of fascia and restoring the ability of muscle tissue to perform multiplanar movements during the next workout or competition.

The human body functions most efficiently when performing movement patterns that coordinate movement between a series of muscles and joints, as opposed to isolation exercises that treat the body as a collection of individual parts. Mobility exercises should be based on how the body is designed to move by using the patterns of hip hinging, squatting, lunging or other single-leg exercises, pushing (both forward and overhead), pulling (both from the front and from overhead), and rotation to take joints through their complete range of motion. Low-intensity mobility exercises can increase circulation and elevate tissue temperature to help remove residual metabolic by-products.

Mobility exercises engage the sensory receptors in both contractile and elastic tissues to fully involve the central nervous system, teaching it positional awareness and how to control the muscle actions that move the entire body. As muscles lengthen, the muscle spindles sense the rate of length change and communicate with motor neurons to initiate muscle contractions. Mobility exercises increase nervous-system activity within muscles, making them more effective at generating force during exercise. Muscle and fascia each contain sensory nerve endings that sense tension, length change, and rate of length change; the multidirectional movements of mobility training help you learn how to feel where your body is in space and how to control its movements.

Establishing more degrees of freedom during joint motion can help improve overall strength while reducing the risk of injury. Tight muscles can restrict joint motion, causing other joints above or below the altered joint to provide the lost motion. Improving the mobility of your hip joints can increase the strength and definition of your hip, thigh, gluteal, lower back, and oblique muscles that connect your legs to your pelvis and your pelvis to your spine; these are often referred to as your core. Mobility exercises for the hip joints allow these muscles to experience a greater range of motion. This can help activate more individual fibers and give you more control while increasing overall strength, both of which can reduce the risk of injury.

Role of Mobility Training

In addition to the muscle and fascia, joint capsules and ligament endings contain numerous sensory receptors that measure and identify pressure, movement, and rate of movement of their respective joints. Mobility exercises that feature slow, controlled movements through a complete range of motion help the nervous system learn how to control movement through the degrees of freedom allowed by each individual joint. Low-intensity contractions that produce low force are essential for recovery; as one set of muscles is contracting to move a limb, the muscles on the opposite side of the joint must lengthen to allow the motion to occur. Known as reciprocal inhibition, this not only helps improve joint motion but also allows your muscles to improve the timing of their contractions and their ability to generate appropriate levels of force to execute efficient, coordinated movement.

Effective mobility workouts use each of the foundational movement patterns as well as combinations of the patterns. Start with slow, controlled linear movements and gradually progress to challenging, fast-paced, multidirectional patterns. Movements with low-intensity resistance could help you move into a deeper and more complete range of motion. If you attend almost any elite or professional-level sporting event early enough to see the pregame warm-up, you will see many of the athletes using these or similar mobility exercises to help them prepare to maximize their performance.

Tools for Mobility

Foam rollers, massage sticks, and percussion guns are all designed specifically for tissue treatment and can help reduce tightness while improving circulation, both of which are essential to the recovery process. These tools apply the principle of autogenic inhibition, which is the exact same principle used by old-fashioned static stretching to increase muscle length. Combining the use of these tools with exercises that require you to move in multiple directions at a variety of different speeds can activate the nervous, circulatory, and respiratory systems responsible for controlling and fueling movement; in other words, it benefits almost all of the systems that control your body.

Mobility training can provide a low-intensity way to recover from a hard or challenging workout the previous day. It also offers a standalone workout when you don't have time for a long workout or just aren't interested in pushing yourself that hard. The following workouts demonstrate different progressions of intensity. On days when you are very sore, using a device like a foam roller, massage stick, or percussion gun to increase tissue temperature, followed by a floor-based mobility workout, can help to reduce overall muscle tightness while elevating tissue temperature, improving both circulation and tissue extensibility, and promoting tissue repair for a more complete recovery.

Massage Stick Workouts

There are different versions of massage sticks, but in general, a massage stick is a long cylinder, between 12 and 24 inches (30 and 61 cm) long, most often with handles that allow the stick to rotate. Some have smooth surfaces, while others have various indentations to increase stimulation. A massage stick is held firmly against a muscle and moved along the line of pull of the fibers; the goal is to use the pressure of the stick to stimulate a release of the Golgi tendon organs for autogenic inhibition while also using the friction to elevate tissue temperatures.

The benefit of using a massage stick is that you can place pressure directly on a spot where a muscle is sore or you feel an adhesion starting to form. The simple yet effective design makes the massage stick ideal for the muscles of the legs, hips, and lower back.

The day after a hard workout, myofascial release can help reduce muscle tension to increase muscle length, but this is a short-term change in the architecture of the tissue. For the best results, once myofascial release has been applied and tissues are lengthened, it is important to move through a range of motion to ensure that the involved muscles can control the change in extensibility and length. This explains why combining tissue treatment with a mobility workout is such an effective recovery strategy the day after a hard workout.

The natural inflammation that occurs during the tissue-repair process, combined with a lack of movement after a hard exercise session, could cause muscle adhesions. As discussed in chapter 5, exercise-induced muscle damage signals the repair process, when new collagen molecules are formed to help repair and strengthen tissue. If tissue is not moved, collagen could bind between layers of muscle. Muscle damage can change the firing patterns of the motor units responsible for muscle contractions as well as the sequence in which muscles are recruited and engaged to produce a movement (MacDonald, Penney, et al. 2013). Using a massage stick (or a foam roller or percussion gun) can help minimize the risk that the new collagen will form adhesions between layers of muscle tissue and will possibly increase the speed of postexercise recovery.

As with a foam roller, when using a massage stick during a warm-up for a normal workout, it is important to use it for only a brief period to elevate tissue temperature and reduce tension. Applying pressure for an extended period could desensitize the muscle and affect its ability to contract during the workout. Think of it this way: You would not want a deep-tissue massage before a workout, because it would relax muscles and limit their ability to produce force. The same is true with a massage stick; too much pressure could reduce the effectiveness of the warm-up. However, the reason why too much myofascial release is dangerous before high-intensity exercise is exactly why it is beneficial after a workout; myofascial release for an extended period after exercise reduces muscle tension and feels very similar to a massage. Limit your use of myofascial release before a workout, but as a component of your recovery program, feel free to use it as long as you feel comfortable.

A massage stick can be used immediately after a workout to support the tissue-repair process or the following day to reduce soreness and the risk of developing adhesions. Remember to apply pressure firmly, moving back and forth over four to six inches (10 to 15 cm) of muscle.

Muscles	Duration	Sets
Calves	45-60 seconds each side	1-3
Adductors and hamstrings	45-60 seconds each side	1-3
Quadriceps	45-60 seconds each side	1-3
Lateral gluteal muscles and piriformis	45-60 seconds each side	1-3
Lower back	45-60 seconds	1-3

Calves

Benefits

Because the calves are responsible both for generating downward force to move over the ground and for receiving ground-reaction forces that are transmitted upward as the feet make contact with the ground, they can take a beating during high-intensity exercise, especially when it involves sprinting, jumping, or making multiple changes of direction. Using a massage stick on the calves can help increase circulation to the muscle tissues while reducing muscle tightness to allow for a normal range of motion from the foot and ankle joints.

Instructions

1. Place your left foot on a bench, jump box, or chair. Hold the massage stick in both hands and press it into the calf muscles just above the back of your ankle.
2. Maintain constant pressure against your muscle tissue as you move the stick up and down vertically. When you feel a tight or sore spot, apply more pressure and move the stick up and down on that spot for 15 to 30 seconds. Switch legs after 45 to 60 seconds.

Correct Your Form

Make sure you are in a comfortable position so that you can apply an appropriate amount of force into your muscle tissue.

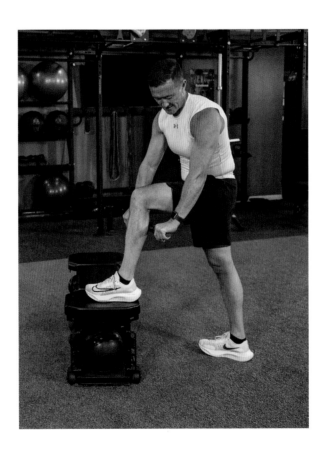

Adductors and Hamstrings

Benefits

The adductor magnus muscles of the upper legs attach to the posterior portion of the femur (that is, the back of the thigh bone). Although the adductors can pull the legs toward the midline of the body, the function they are designed to perform is to move the legs forward and backward. When the right leg is in front of the body, the right adductor magnus will pull it backward into extension. When the right leg is behind the body, the adductor magnus will pull it forward into flexion. Because these muscles are always working when a person runs, they can experience a tremendous amount of stress during high-intensity running workouts. If the adductors become too tight or fatigued from overuse, they could change the function of the joints above and below—the hip and knee, respectively. Using a massage stick can help reduce muscle tightness and allow these muscles to function to the best of their ability.

The hamstrings work with the adductor group to help extend the hip and control stability of the knee; excessive tightness in the hamstrings could restrict range of motion of the hip and reduce stability of the knee. Because the adductors and hamstrings lie next to one another, a massage stick can be used on both areas at the same time to improve tissue extensibility, which can help ensure that the hip can remain mobile and functional in all three planes of motion while effectively stabilizing the knee.

Instructions

1. Place your left heel on a bench, jump box, or chair while keeping your knee relatively straight. Hold the massage stick along the inside of the thigh and pull it toward your thigh bone to apply maximal pressure.

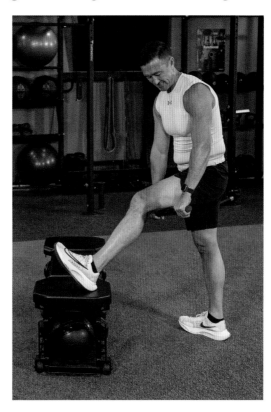

2. Maintain constant pressure against your muscle tissue as you move the stick up and down vertically. When you feel a tight or sore spot, apply more pressure and move the stick up and down on that spot for 15 to 30 seconds. Switch legs after 45 to 60 seconds.

3. To reduce tightness in the hamstrings, place more pressure on the back of the leg. To improve tissue extensibility of the adductors, put more pressure on the inside of the thigh.

Correct Your Form

Hold the massage stick tightly and press it firmly into the back of your thigh as you move it back and forth to create pressure.

Quadriceps

Benefits

In most sports, the quadriceps muscles can experience heavy eccentric loading and high amounts of force during rapid changes of direction, which could cause DOMS. Using a massage stick on the quadriceps immediately after and the day after exercise can help improve circulation so that the metabolic by-products associated with DOMS can be removed more quickly. In addition, reducing tension in the quadriceps can lower stress on the knee joint, allowing it to function more effectively.

Instructions

1. Place your left foot on a bench, jump box, or chair so that your left leg is relatively straight. Hold the massage stick in both hands and press it into the top of the thigh muscles just above your knee (a).

2. Maintain constant pressure against your muscle tissue as you press the massage stick into the muscle while moving it back and forth vertically. Move the stick up and down along the front, inside, and outside of the thigh to reduce tension in all four muscles that comprise the quadriceps (b). When you feel a tight or sore spot, apply more pressure and move the stick up and down on that spot for 15 to 30 seconds. Switch legs after 45 to 60 seconds.

Correct Your Form

The quadriceps helps extend the knee and straighten the leg. Placing your foot on an elevated object such as a bench, jump box, or chair allows you to keep your leg relatively straight so you can apply pressure to all four muscles that comprise the quadriceps, which is one way to make this stretch more effective.

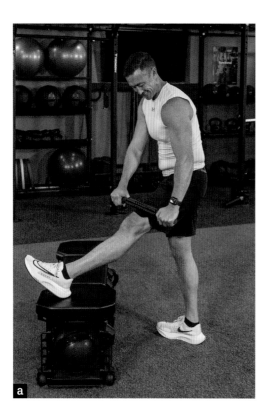

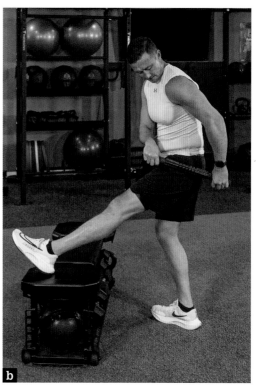

Lateral Gluteal Muscles and Piriformis

Benefits

The gluteal complex (often called the glutes) includes the gluteus minimus, medius, and ever-popular maximus. All three muscles help produce external rotation of the hip; when these muscles become too tight, they could change the position and function of the knee joint. Using a massage stick to reduce pressure in these muscles can help ensure optimal hip function and knee position.

Instructions

1. Place your left heel on a bench, jump box, or chair while keeping your knee extended and your leg relatively straight. Hold the massage stick in both hands and pull it into the large muscles on the outside of your glutes and thigh.

2. Maintain constant pressure against your muscle tissue as you move the stick up and down vertically. When you feel a tight or sore spot, apply more pressure and move the stick up and down on that spot for 15 to 30 seconds. Switch legs after 45 to 60 seconds.

Correct Your Form

For best results, keep the pressure on the outside portion of the back of the leg and lower gluteal complex.

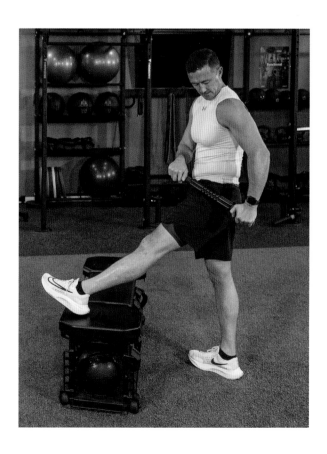

Lower Back

Benefits

The muscles of the lower back help to control the position of the pelvis and movement of the spine. When these muscles become too tight, they could pull upward on the pelvis and create an anterior pelvic tilt that changes the range of motion of the hip joints. Reducing tightness in the lower back muscles can help reduce discomfort while allowing the hips to function to the best of their ability.

Instructions

1. Stand with your spine long and your feet about hip-width apart. Hold the massage stick in both hands and pull it into the muscles of your lower back, just above the back of your pelvis.
2. Maintain constant pressure against your muscle tissue as you move the stick up and down vertically. When you feel a tight or sore spot, apply more pressure and move the stick up and down on that spot for 15 to 30 seconds. Maintain steady pressure for 45 to 60 seconds.

Correct Your Form

Keep your spine tall and your feet firmly planted into the ground so that you can apply the greatest amount of pressure to the muscles.

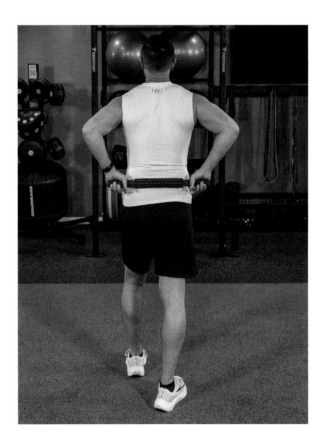

Percussion Gun Workouts

A percussion gun can be used both to prepare muscle tissue before a workout and to reduce muscular tension and facilitate the return to homeostasis once the workout is over. When using a percussion gun as a component of a warm-up, if possible, use it on a lower frequency for 30 seconds or less. The goal is to activate the muscle spindles so the muscles can contract at a faster velocity. Holding a gun on a muscle for too long could stimulate autogenic inhibition, causing a muscle to relax and lengthen, which is not ideal before a workout. Once a workout is over, or the day following a hard workout when you're very sore, using a percussion gun set to a higher frequency for a longer period of time can feel like a massage without the expense or hassle of a trip to the spa.

Move the gun at a slow, steady pace, approximately one inch (2.54 cm) per second, for a total of 30 to 60 seconds for each body part. When you feel a tight or sore spot, hold the gun on that location for 5 to 10 seconds. There is no need to press hard into the muscle; simply let the weight of the gun apply the pressure. Focus on applying the pressure of the gun to muscles and soft tissues. It is best to avoid bony surfaces and joint structures.

Muscles	Duration	Sets
Bottom of feet	45-60 seconds each side	1-3
Calves	45-60 seconds each side	1-3
Hamstrings	45-60 seconds each side	1-3
Adductors	45-60 seconds each side	1-3
Quadriceps	45-60 seconds each side	1-3
Latissimus dorsi	45-60 seconds each side	1-3
Pectoralis major	45-60 seconds each side	1-3
Biceps	45-60 seconds each side	1-3
Forearms	45-60 seconds each side	1-3

Bottom of Feet

Benefits

There are 26 different bones in the feet. When the muscle tissue becomes overly tight, it could affect how the bones work together to allow mobility when the foot hits the ground before converting to stability as the foot pushes off the ground for the next phase of the gait cycle. Reducing tightness in the muscles in the bottom of the foot helps to ensure optimal function during movement.

Instructions

1. Sit in a cross-leg position with the bottom of your left foot resting on your right knee.
2. Apply light pressure from the gun to the muscles along the bottom of the foot. Once you hit a tight spot, hold the pressure for 5 to 10 seconds before moving to another spot. Maintain pressure for 45 to 60 seconds on each foot.

Correct Your Form

If possible, use a flat or ball-shaped head on the percussion gun; a pointed head may apply too much pressure to specific spots. Try to keep your foot in a fully dorsiflexed position so the muscles are lengthened; this can help to ensure optimal benefits for reducing muscle tightness.

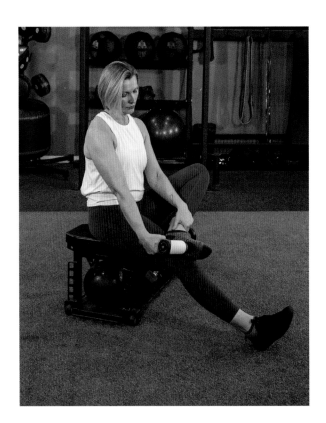

Calves

Benefits

As a result of pushing force into the ground while lifting, running, or jumping, the calf muscles are used frequently during high-intensity exercise. This frequent use means that the muscle cells are constantly producing both adenosine triphosphate and metabolic by-products; applying pressure from a percussion gun can help to increase circulation in an effort to promote a complete return to homeostasis.

Instructions

1. Place your right foot on a bench, jump box, or chair. Hold the percussion gun lightly against the calf muscles just above the back of your ankle.

2. Maintain light but constant pressure against your muscle tissue as you move the gun up and down vertically between your ankle and just below the back of your knee. Once you locate a tight or sore spot, maintain pressure on that spot for 5 to 10 seconds. Switch legs after 45 to 60 seconds.

Correct Your Form

Move the percussion gun all around the muscle tissue, both up and down and side to side. The goal is to apply the gun to as much of the tissue as possible. There is no need to press the head of the gun deep into the muscle tissue; simply hold it against the surface of the skin and let it do the work.

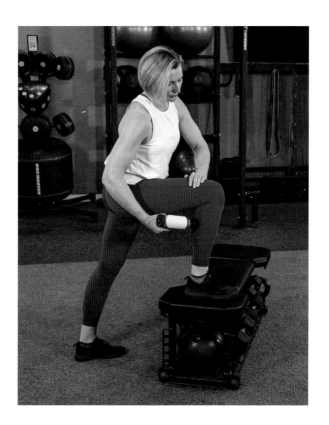

Hamstrings

Benefits

The hamstrings help extend the hip and maintain stability of the knee. These muscles also help to decelerate forward motion of the hip and knee during fast-paced running; thus, they can experience tremendous amounts of force that results in metabolic by-products becoming stuck in the muscle tissue. This helps to explain why the hamstrings can be more sore than other muscles the day after playing sports. A percussion gun helps to improve tissue extensibility while facilitating the return to homeostasis to ensure that the hamstrings can effectively recover from one workout and be prepared for the next.

Instructions

1. Place your left heel on a bench, jump box, or chair while keeping your knee extended and your leg relatively straight. Hold the percussion gun in one hand and place it against the muscles along the back of the thigh.

2. Maintain constant pressure against your muscle tissue as you move the gun up and down vertically. When you feel a sore spot, apply light pressure and hold the gun on that location for 5 to 10 seconds. Switch legs after 45 to 60 seconds.

Correct Your Form

Because the hamstrings help flex the knee, keeping your leg mostly straight with your knee extended places the muscles in a lengthened position for the best possible results while using the percussion gun.

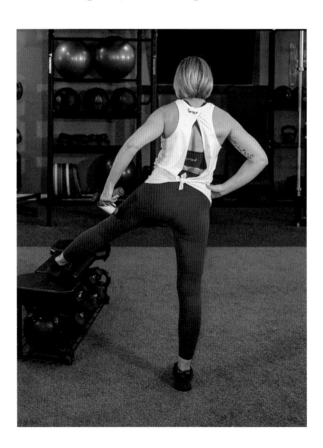

Adductors

Benefits

When the adductors become too tight or fatigued from overuse, they could change the function of the hip and knee joints. Using a percussion gun after a workout can help reduce muscle tightness while promoting circulation to allow these muscles to completely return to homeostasis.

Instructions

1. Place your right heel on a bench, jump box, or chair while keeping your knee relatively straight. Hold the percussion gun along the inside of the thigh and move it vertically between your knee and hip joint.

2. Maintain constant pressure against your muscle tissue as you move the percussion gun up and down vertically. When you feel a tight or sore spot, apply more pressure on that location for 5 to 10 seconds. Switch legs after 45 to 60 seconds.

Correct Your Form

There is no need to press the gun deep into the muscle tissue; simply hold the percussion gun against the muscles as you move it up and down along the inside of your thigh.

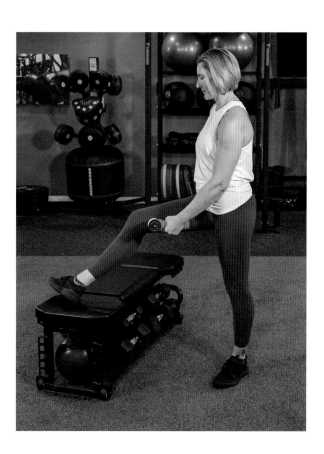

Quadriceps

Benefits

During high-intensity activities, the quadriceps muscles can experience large amounts of force that ultimately result in DOMS the day after a workout. Using a percussion gun on these muscles can help improve circulation to facilitate the return to homeostasis so that the muscles can be fully prepared for the next hard workout or competition.

Instructions

1. Place your left foot on a bench, jump box, or chair so that your left knee is bent at approximately 90 degrees. This will place the muscles in a lengthened position; applying pressure from a percussion gun while muscles are lengthened can help facilitate tissue release and improve extensibility. Hold the percussion gun lightly against your muscle tissue and allow the weight of the gun to create pressure as you move it along the front of your thigh muscles.

2. Maintain constant pressure against your muscle tissue as you hold the gun lightly against your thigh and move it back and forth between the top of the knee and the bottom of the hip. (Avoid letting the percussion gun hit your kneecaps.) When you feel a tight or sore spot, apply steady pressure on that location for 5 to 10 seconds. Switch legs after 45 to 60 seconds.

Correct Your Form

The quadriceps muscle helps extend the knee and straighten the leg. Keeping your knee bent so that you can apply pressure to the muscle while it is in a lengthened position is one way to make this stretch more effective.

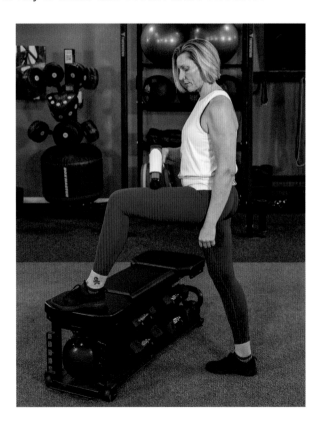

Latissimus Dorsi

Benefits

The attachments of the latissimus dorsi on the humeral bones of the upper arms can create internal rotation at the glenohumeral joints of the shoulders. When this muscle is too tight, it can pull the shoulders forward, which could restrict the range of motion of the glenohumeral joints. Using the gun to reduce tightness of the latissimus dorsi along the side of the rib cage under the arm could help to reduce overall tightness, promote recovery, and restore optimal mobility at the shoulders.

Instructions

1. Raise your left arm into the air (this can be done seated or standing) and place your left hand on the back of your head; this will increase tension on the latissimus dorsi muscle. Hold the percussion gun in your right hand so that the head of the gun is pointed toward you. Place the head against the thick part of the muscle, just below your left armpit.

2. Maintain gentle but steady pressure against your muscle tissue as you move the gun up and down along the outer edge of the rib cage vertically. When you feel a tight or sore spot, apply steady pressure on that location for 5 to 10 seconds. Switch sides after 45 to 60 seconds.

Correct Your Form

Keep the head of the percussion gun on the muscle tissue. Avoid letting it hit the rib cage.

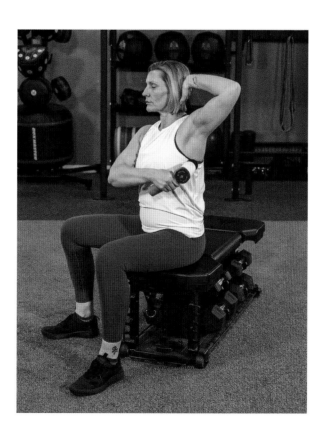

Pectoralis Major

Benefits

The pectoralis major connects the humeral bones of the upper arms to the sternum of the chest. When this muscle becomes tight from overuse, it can cause internal rotation of the shoulders, which restricts the range of motion and could cause discomfort in the upper back. It can be difficult to use a foam roller or massage stick to perform myofascial release on the front of the upper body, especially the chest, which may make the percussion gun the most effective tool for this muscle.

Instructions

1. From a seated, standing, or lying position, let your right hand hang by your side or rest in your lap. Hold the percussion gun in your left hand so that the head is pointed toward you. Apply the gun to the muscle tissue between your shoulder and chest.

2. Maintain gentle but steady pressure against your muscle tissue as you move the gun back and forth between your chest and shoulder. When you feel a tight or sore spot, apply steady pressure on that location for 5 to 10 seconds. Switch sides after 45 to 60 seconds.

Correct Your Form

Holding the shoulder in an externally rotated position lengthens the muscle tissue for a greater response. Focus on keeping the gun on muscle tissue; try to avoid hitting your chest or upper arm bones.

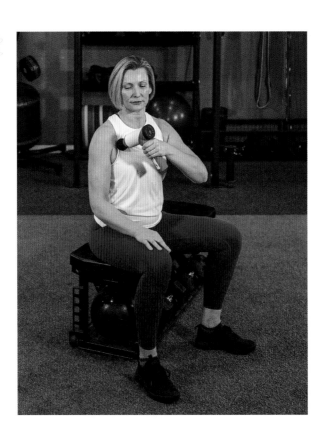

Biceps

Benefits

The biceps muscles not only flex the elbow but also help with controlling motion of the shoulder joints. When these muscles become tight from overuse, they can pull the shoulders forward, which could restrict range of motion and result in back pain. Reducing tension in the biceps helps to promote tissue repair while ensuring optimal function of both the elbow and the shoulder.

Instructions

1. From a seated position, let your right arm rest on your lap so that your elbow is bent. Hold the percussion gun in your left hand so the head is pointed toward your arm muscles. Apply the gun to the thick muscle tissue between your elbow and shoulder.

2. Maintain gentle but steady pressure against your muscle tissue as you move the gun back and forth between your elbow and shoulder. When you feel a tight or sore spot, apply steady pressure on that location for 5 to 10 seconds. Switch sides after 45 to 60 seconds.

Correct Your Form

To increase the stretch, allow your arm to hang fully straight (lengthening the biceps) while using the percussion gun.

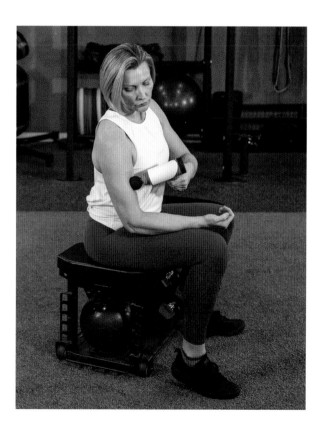

Forearms

Benefits

As a result of high-intensity strength training using barbells, dumbbells, kettlebells, or any other piece of equipment that requires a tight grip, the muscles of the wrist and forearm can take a beating and become excessively tight. Reducing tension in forearm muscles could help to maintain optimal force production while reducing the risk of developing overuse injuries such as carpal tunnel syndrome or lateral epicondylitis (tennis elbow) in your wrist and elbow, respectively.

Instructions

1. For the flexor muscles that feel tight as a result of gripping (a weight or a phone): Hold your left arm in your lap so that the palm of your left hand is facing up toward the ceiling. Hold the percussion gun in your right hand so that the head is pointed toward your left forearm muscles. Apply the gun to the thick muscle tissue between your wrist and elbow (a).

2. For the extensor muscles that feel tight from typing: Hold your right arm in your lap so that the palm of your right hand is facing down. Hold the percussion gun in your left hand so that the head is resting on the top of your forearm muscles (b). Allow the weight of the gun to apply pressure as you slowly move the gun back and forth over the thick part of the muscle at the top of your forearm.

3. Maintain gentle but steady pressure against your muscle tissue as you move the gun back and forth between your wrist and elbow. When you feel a tight or sore spot, apply steady pressure on that location for 5 to 10 seconds. Switch sides after 45 to 60 seconds.

Correct Your Form

Focus on keeping the head of the percussion gun against the muscle tissue; try to avoid letting it hit the bones of your elbow and wrist.

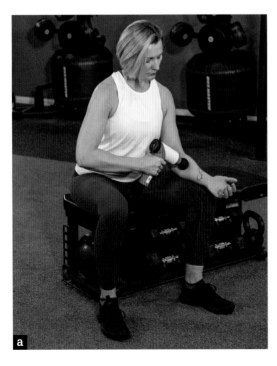
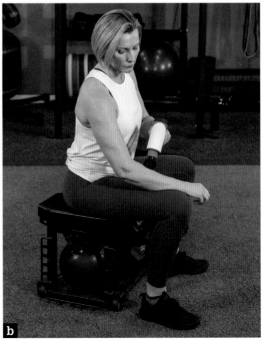

Static Stretching Workouts

Static stretches are the same ones you did as a kid when you were told to run two laps and circle up before a sport practice. Static stretching uses the principle of autogenic inhibition to reduce tightness and allow a muscle to lengthen. There are two ways to manipulate static stretching to increase the stretch effect:

1. When stretching a muscle, contracting its functional antagonist, or the muscle that performs the opposite function (the antagonist for the hamstrings in the back of the thigh is the quadriceps in the front of the thigh, for example), can help to reduce neural drive and tension, allowing the muscle to achieve a greater length. For example, when doing a standing hamstring stretch, contracting the quadriceps can inhibit the hamstrings to allow them to experience a greater stretch.

2. Holding a muscle in a lengthened position and then contracting it for four to six seconds before relaxing it can allow it to lengthen and move the joint into a deeper range of motion. For example, when doing the wall calf stretch, pushing your back foot into the ground—like pointing your toes—for four to six seconds, then relaxing and moving to a new range of motion, can allow you to achieve a deeper stretch and greater range of motion from your ankle.

Because the purpose of autogenic inhibition (static stretching) is to lengthen muscles by reducing tightness, it is not advised to do this before a workout. Instead, for best results, save static stretching for after a workout or the following day, when you want to reduce soreness and restore or enhance joint motion.

Exercise	Duration	Sets
Wall calf stretch	45-60 seconds each side	1-3
Wall quadriceps stretch	45-60 seconds each side	1-3
Wall chest stretch	45-60 seconds each side	1-3
Wall latissimus dorsi stretch	45-60 seconds each side	1-3
Standing hamstring stretch	45-60 seconds each side	1-3
Standing adductor stretch	45-60 seconds each side	1-3
Standing hip flexor stretch	45-60 seconds each side	1-3
Standing biceps stretch	45-60 seconds	1-3

Wall Calf Stretch

Benefits

Whether walking, running, lifting, or simply standing, the calf muscles are constantly working. When they become overly tight, they can restrict motion in both the ankle and hip. This stretch lengthens the muscles of the lower leg to allow for optimal mobility of the ankle and hip.

Instructions

1. Stand facing a wall or solid object (such as a squat cage). Place your left foot in front of your body close to the wall and lean your body weight forward, into the wall, as you extend your right leg behind you while pushing your right heel into the ground.

2. To increase the stretch, press the ball of your right foot into the ground (like stepping on an accelerator) for four to six seconds. Relax, then lean farther forward while keeping your right heel pushed down; if necessary, slide your right heel backward a bit to increase the length. Hold this new length for 15 to 20 seconds before repeating the contraction.

3. Repeat the contract–relax cycle for a total of 45 to 60 seconds, then switch legs.

Correct Your Form

Take a deep breath while you are contracting your calf muscles by pressing your foot into the ground, then exhale as you relax and move deeper into the stretch.

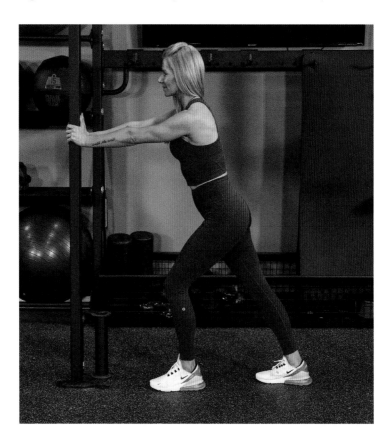

Wall Quadriceps Stretch

Benefits

This stretch can reduce tightness and promote blood flow in the large quadriceps muscles of the thigh, which helps to maintain optimal hip mobility.

Instructions

1. Stand up tall with your feet hip-width apart. If necessary, position yourself near a wall or solid object for support.

2. Bring the top of your left foot up so that it is resting in your left hand as you pull your left heel closer to your glutes. Hold for 10 to 15 seconds, then press the top of your left foot into your hand like you're trying to straighten your leg (but don't let go). Hold for 4 to 6 seconds, release, then pull your heel closer to your tailbone and hold for 10 to 15 seconds. Repeat for a total of 45 to 60 seconds, then switch legs.

Correct Your Form

Take deep breaths while stretching. Inhale while extending your leg, then exhale as you pull your heel closer to your glutes to increase the stretch.

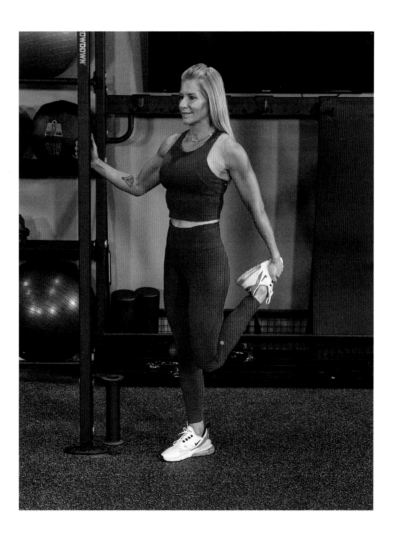

Wall Chest Stretch

Benefits

This stretch can help loosen the chest and shoulder muscles, which can become tight from exercises such as chest presses and flys but can often also be shortened as a result of spending hours using a computer or phone. Stretching the muscles in the chest and along the front of the body can reduce stress through the upper back and shoulders.

Instructions

1. Stand with the wall to your right side, about an arm's length away. Place your right hand against the wall so that your fingers are pointed behind you.

2. Press your right hand into the wall and extend your left arm as you turn to your left to increase the stretch on the chest muscles. Hold the stretch for 10 to 15 seconds, then press your hand into the wall and contract your chest muscles for 4 to 6 seconds. Take a deep breath, and as you exhale, move to the new range of motion. Repeat for a total of 45 to 60 seconds, then switch sides.

Correct Your Form

Stretch to a point of mild tension. Try to avoid stretching too deeply; that could lengthen the muscle beyond its ability, potentially causing injury. Breathe deeply while holding the stretch. Attempt to go a little farther into the range of motion with each exhale.

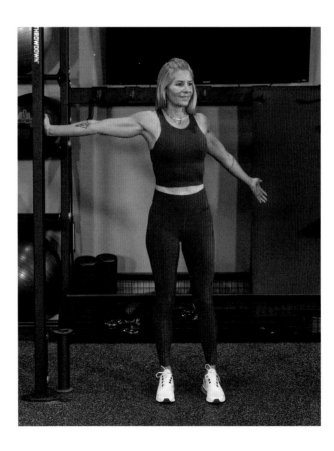

Wall Latissimus Dorsi Stretch

Benefits

The large latissimus dorsi muscle can be sore the day after a hard upper-body workout or playing a sport that involves a lot of upper-body movements such as throwing or swinging a racket. Using a wall helps to increase leverage and stretch into the muscle tissue.

Instructions

1. Stand next to the wall so that it is on your right side. Extend your right arm overhead and place your right elbow against the wall. To increase the stretch, move your feet farther from the wall and stagger them so that the right foot is forward.

2. Extend your right arm as you lean against your elbow for 10 to 15 seconds, then push your elbow into the wall while contracting your latissimus dorsi muscle. Hold for 4 to 6 seconds, take a deep breath in, and as you exhale, allow yourself to sink deeper into the stretch. Repeat for a total of 45 to 60 seconds, then switch sides.

Correct Your Form

Moving your feet farther from the wall can increase the stretch effect on your upper back. Breathe comfortably during the exercise. On each exhale, allow yourself to sink deeper into the stretch.

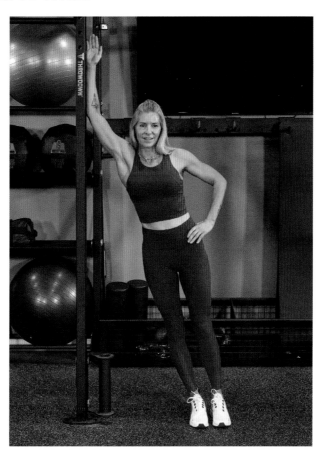

Standing Hamstring Stretch

Benefits

The hamstrings work to both flex (bend) the knee and extend the hip (moving the leg behind the body), which means they can take a beating during many high-intensity workouts or sports that require rapid acceleration and deceleration. Static stretching helps to reduce tightness by increasing the length of the muscle. The contract–relax cycle can help the muscle to relax while improving circulation for optimal recovery.

Instructions

1. Stand with your feet approximately hip-width apart. Extend your right leg straight in front of you so that it is resting on your right heel while you place both hands on the top of your left thigh.

2. Sink back into your hips while keeping the knee fully extended and the leg straight to increase the overall stretch. Hold for 10 to 15 seconds, then press the back of your right heel down into the ground (to activate your hamstrings) for 4 to 6 seconds. Exhale as you relax the muscles and sink deeper into the stretch. Repeat for a total of 45 to 60 seconds, then switch legs.

Correct Your Form

The hamstrings help to extend the hip and flex the knee. To stretch these muscles, make sure the knee is fully extended and the leg is straight. Breathe comfortably during the stretch; each time you exhale, sink back deeper into your hips to increase the stretch on the muscles.

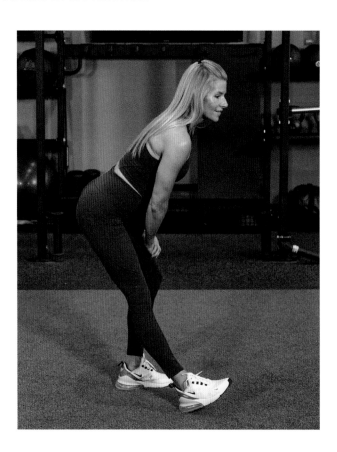

Standing Adductor Stretch

Benefits

The adductors are responsible for flexing and extending the hips and can experience a lot of force during sprints and rapid changes of direction. Stretching the adductors can reduce tightness to maintain optimal hip mobility. This is a great stretch when the legs are sore the day after a game or match that required a lot of starting and stopping while running.

Instructions

1. Stand with your feet wider than shoulder-width apart so that your right foot is slightly more forward than your left (the heel of your right foot should line up with the toes of your left). Extend your left leg directly out to your left so your entire left foot is flat on the ground.

2. Press your left heel into the ground and shift your hips to the right as you keep your spine long. Breathe deeply and exhale as you focus your gaze straight ahead; hold for 10 to 15 seconds. Take a deep breath in, squeeze your left gluteal muscles, and push your left heel into the ground for 4 to 6 seconds, then exhale as you shift farther to your right into a deeper range of motion. Hold for 10 to 15 seconds and repeat for a total of 45 to 60 seconds. Switch sides.

Correct Your Form

Keep your spine long and rotate both shoulders when turning into the stretch. Breathe deeply while stretching; try to move into a deeper stretch and new range of motion with each exhale.

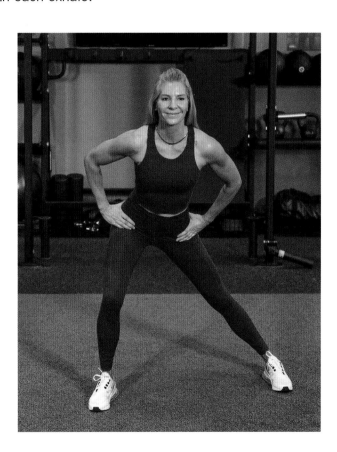

Standing Hip Flexor Stretch

Benefits

The hip flexors can become tight from spending too much time in a seated position. Add in high-intensity exercises for the legs and it is easy to understand why the hips and lower back might be sore the day after a hard workout or competition. By lengthening and relaxing the muscles responsible for flexing the hips, this stretch helps to reduce stress on the lower back while promoting optimal hip mobility.

Instructions

1. Stand with your feet about shoulder-width apart and rotate your right foot inward to point toward your left foot. Roll your pelvis backward (like tucking your tailbone under your hips). Keep your spine long, and extend your right arm directly overhead.

2. Lean back slightly while also leaning to your left (you should feel the stretch directly in the front of your right hip). Hold the stretch for 10 to 15 seconds before pressing your right heel down and squeezing your right glutes for 4 to 6 seconds. As you relax your right leg, exhale deeply and sink back deeper into the stretch. Repeat for a total of 45 to 60 seconds, then switch legs.

Correct Your Form

Keeping your spine long and your pelvis tucked under will help to increase the stretch on these deep muscles, whereas leaning back and to the side takes the stretch deeper for a greater range of motion.

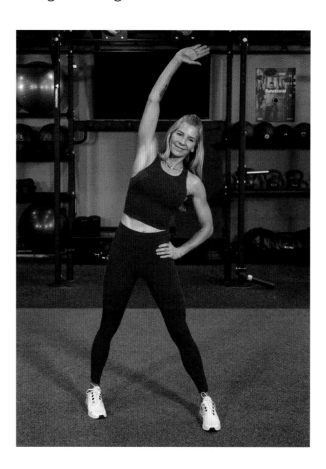

Standing Biceps Stretch

Benefits

When overly tight, the biceps muscles can pull the scapulae forward and restrict mobility of the shoulder joints. Reducing tension in the biceps helps to ensure optimal function of the shoulders.

Instructions

1. Stand with your feet hip-width apart and your knees slightly bent (this stretch can also be done from a seated position). Raise your chest, keep your spine long, and hold both arms straight out to the sides with your palms facing the ground.

2. Take a deep breath in. As you exhale, point backward with your fingers while lifting your chest, like a flight attendant pointing to the window exits at the rear of an airplane. Continue to breathe deeply and move your arms into a deeper range of motion with each exhale. Hold for a total of 45 to 60 seconds.

Correct Your Form

Keep your spine long with your chest raised to increase the stretch on your biceps muscles.

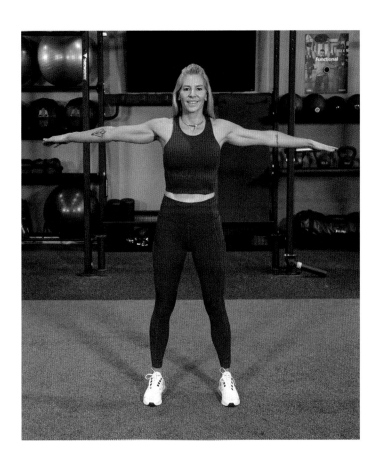

Ground-Based Workouts

The purpose of low-intensity mobility exercises is to elevate your heart rate and increase circulation to deliver new oxygen and nutrients while removing metabolites from the involved muscles. A secondary benefit is to maintain or enhance joint function by moving your limbs through their complete range of motion. This is essential, especially when you are sore from a very hard workout. In addition, performing these mobility exercises when you are sore can help you learn how to work through discomfort and establish a positive mindset of "I can do this."

Because these exercises are supported by the floor, they reduce the load of gravity on your body and are perfect for when you are very sore but want to move and work through the soreness to flush your muscles.

The following are two options for using these exercises. Both will work, but vertical loading can increase the intensity by removing the rest interval between exercises; this is recommended if you want to feel like you're doing a bit of a workout while focusing on your recovery.

1. Horizontal loading is completing all sets of a given exercise before moving on to the next.
2. Vertical loading (also known as circuit training) is moving from one exercise to the next with minimal rest and completing the assigned number of exercises as a function of completing the circuit.

Exercise	Duration or repetitions	Sets
Gluteal bridges	12-20 repetitions	1-3
Side-lying quadriceps stretch	3-5 repetitions, 45-60 seconds each side	1-3
90-90 hamstring stretch with leg straightening	3-5 repetitions, 45-60 seconds each side	1-3
Upward facing dog	30-45 seconds	1-3
Child's pose with palms up	30-45 seconds	1-3
Seated cross-leg rotation	30-45 seconds each side	1-3
Pigeon pose	30-45 seconds each side	1-3
Plank with hip extension and arm rotation	6-10 repetitions each side	1-3

Gluteal Bridges

Benefits

Because the gluteus maximus is the primary muscle responsible for extending the hips and moving the lower body, the glutes and hip flexors take a lot of abuse during high-intensity exercise, and as a result, they could experience both tightness from overuse and DOMS from metabolic by-products in the muscle cells. Using the glutes in this exercise can help stretch the hip flexors while improving circulation in the glutes. After spending a long time in a seated position, this exercise is an excellent dynamic stretch that can help reduce tightness and restore range of motion in the hips; the more mobility there is in the hips, the better it is for the lower back.

Instructions

1. Lie on your back so your feet are flat on the floor with your knees pointed up to the ceiling; your feet should be about 18 inches (46 cm) or so away from your glutes. Keep your arms along your sides with your palms rotated up to face the ceiling (this helps stretch your shoulder muscles). Pull your toes up toward your shins so that you are resting on the heels of both feet (a).

2. To perform the exercise, press your heels down as you squeeze your glutes and lift your hips toward the ceiling (b). (Think about squeezing a coin between your gluteal muscles to increase the muscle activation.) Push up for a count of 1 or 2 seconds, then lower for a count of 3 or 4 seconds. Complete 12 to 20 repetitions. If you are feeling good, do more repetitions; if you are feeling sore, do less.

Correct Your Form

If you notice your hamstring muscles along the backs of your thighs cramping, then your feet are too close to your hips; simply move your feet forward a little. If you feel discomfort in your lower back, then your feet are too far away; move them back toward your tailbone. Focusing on squeezing your glutes will help increase circulation and the stretch response in the hip flexors.

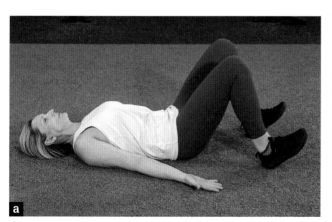
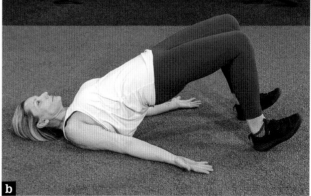

Side-Lying Quadriceps Stretch

Benefits

The large quadriceps muscles of the leg are used during running and lower-body strength training. This stretch can help reduce overall tightness, promote blood flow, and support optimal mobility of the hips.

Instructions

1. Lie on your right side so that your left leg is stacked on top of your right; place your right forearm on the floor so that you can support your upper-body weight.

2. Hold the top of your left foot in your left hand while pulling your left heel closer to your glutes. Hold for 10 to 15 seconds, then press the top of your left foot into your hand like you're trying to straighten your leg (but don't let go). Hold for 4 to 6 seconds. Release, then pull your heel closer to your tailbone and hold for 10 to 15 seconds. Repeat for a total of 45 to 60 seconds, then switch legs.

Correct Your Form

Take deep breaths while stretching. Inhale while extending your leg, then exhale as you pull your heel closer to your glutes to increase the stretch.

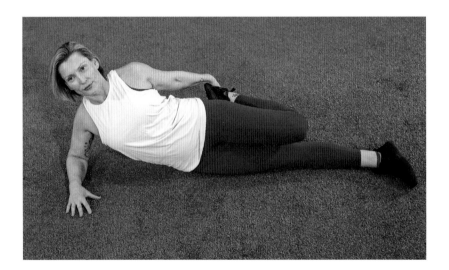

90-90 Hamstring Stretch With Leg Straightening

Benefits

Improving flexibility and hip mobility can reduce muscular tightness and alleviate discomfort in the lower back. Contracting the quadriceps sends a signal to the hamstrings to allow them to lengthen and relax in order for the knee to fully extend.

Instructions

1. Lie flat on your back with the legs next to one another. Pick up your right leg and pull your knee toward your chest while placing your right hand behind your right knee and your left hand on top of the knee (*a*).

2. Allow the left leg to remain flat on the floor while you keep a 90-degree bend in your right knee; pull your right knee back toward your chest (to increase the stretch, press the back of your left leg into the floor). Hold the stretch for 10 to 15 seconds, then extend your right leg as straight as possible while squeezing the muscles of your right thigh for 4 to 6 seconds (*b*). (This sends the signal to the hamstrings to relax and lengthen.) Take a deep breath, and as you exhale, relax the right leg and move it back into the stretch with the knee at 90 degrees. Repeat for a total of 45 to 60 seconds with the right leg before switching legs.

Correct Your Form

To increase the stretch, make sure to extend your knee so that it is fully straight. If the knee remains slightly bent, the hamstrings will not be in an extended, lengthened position. Continue to breathe deeply during the exercise; exhale as you move your bent leg toward your chest and inhale as you straighten your leg.

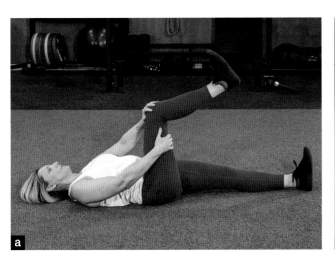

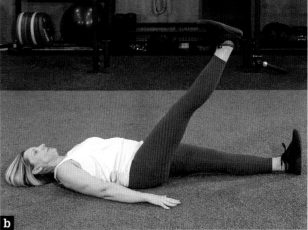

Upward Facing Dog

Benefits

Remaining in a seated position for too long can cause the hip flexor, quadriceps, and abdominal muscles to become tight and restrict motion at the hips and lower back, especially during the recovery process when they are still working to repair and remove all of the metabolic by-products. This move can help lengthen the muscles along the front of the body to ensure optimal posture and motion of the hip joints.

Instructions

1. Lie prone (face down) on the ground with your legs extended, your hands directly under your shoulders, your upper arms next to your rib cage, and your elbows pointed toward your feet.
2. Press your hands into the ground to lift your chest and the fronts of your legs off the ground, creating full extension of the spine.
3. To increase the intensity of the stretch, squeeze your glutes while pressing your hips down. Hold for 30 to 45 seconds before lowering to the ground.

Correct Your Form

As you press your hips down, think about lifting your chest and lengthening through the front of your body. Only go to a comfortable range of motion; do not try to force a backward bend of the spine. Practice squeezing your glutes while lifting only your chest off the ground if holding your entire body up is too challenging.

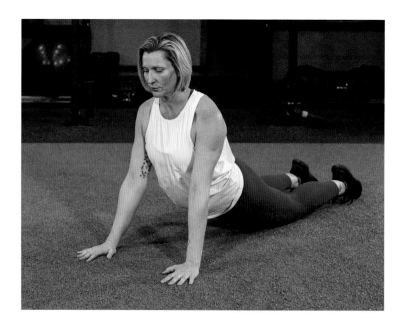

Child's Pose With Palms Up

Benefits

This move can reduce tension and tightness in the upper back muscles. Rotating the palms to face upward can increase the stretch effect and help improve the range of motion of the shoulder joints.

Instructions

1. Kneel with your feet tucked under your body. As you sink your rear end back over your heels, reach both arms straight out in front of your body and turn your hands up so that both palms are facing the ceiling.
2. Take a deep breath. As you exhale, open up your knees and sink deeper into your hips; hold for 30 to 45 seconds.

Correct Your Form

Allow your legs to spread open as you sink your weight down into your glutes. Breathe deeply, and on each exhale, try to sink back deeper to increase the stretch.

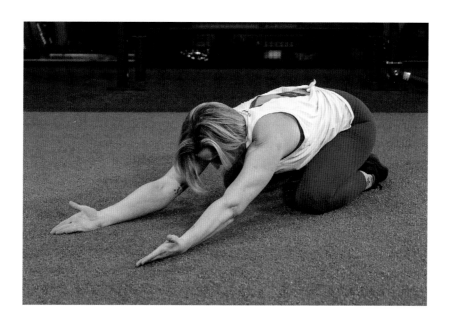

Seated Cross-Leg Rotation

Benefits

This move improves the mobility and range of motion of the thoracic spine by stretching the chest and the core muscles that control trunk rotation.

Instructions

1. Sit down with both legs extended straight in front of you. Pick up your right leg and cross it over the left so that your right foot is flat on the ground and your right knee is pointed toward the ceiling.

2. Rotate your upper body all the way to your right and place your left arm on the outside of your right leg. Place your right arm behind your body to help increase leverage. Hold the stretch for 10 to 15 seconds, then push your left arm into your right leg and try to rotate farther to your right for 4 to 6 seconds. Take a deep breath, and as you exhale, relax and move into a deeper range of motion. Repeat for a total of 30 to 45 seconds before switching sides.

Correct Your Form

Keep your spine long and straight to ensure an optimal range of motion. Breathe deeply; as you exhale, relax and move deeper into the range of motion of the stretch.

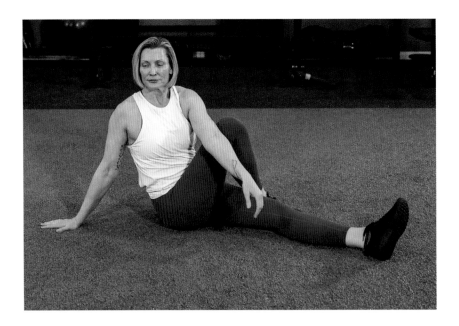

Pigeon Pose

Benefits

This is a yoga move that can help improve hip mobility and reduce tightness in the lower back.

Instructions

1. Start in a seated position with both legs crossed in front of you. Keep your right leg bent and in front of your body as you straighten your left leg and place it so that it is pointed directly behind you.

2. Keep your hands to your sides for support as you hinge forward from your waist to lower your chest closer to your right leg. Hold for 10 to 15 seconds, then press the front of your left thigh into the floor for 4 to 6 seconds. Exhale and relax to move into a deeper range of motion. Repeat for a total of 30 to 45 seconds, then switch legs.

Correct Your Form

If the knee of your straight leg (the left leg in the example above) cannot touch the ground, use a rolled towel or yoga block to create that point of contact (this is important for the contract–relax cycle of the stretch). Breathe comfortably; with each exhale, move into a deeper range of motion.

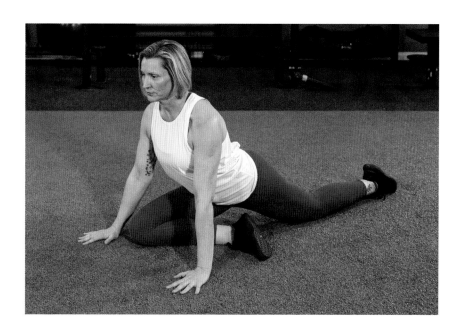

Plank With Hip Extension and Arm Rotation

Benefits

The core muscles connect the hips to the shoulders. This is a great mobility exercise for stretching the hip flexors and opening up the hips while improving motion in the thoracic spine. The upward rotation of the arm helps to increase the stretch response in the opposite hip.

Instructions

1. Start in a high-plank position with the hands directly under the shoulders and the feet in line with the hips. Bring your right knee forward to the outside of the right elbow and place your right foot on the outside of your right hand while pushing back through your left heel to straighten the left leg (a). This helps increase the stretch in the left hip flexor.

2. Use your right hand to reach under your left shoulder (b), then rotate to your right and reach up toward the ceiling while pushing back with your left heel (c). Keep your spine straight by bracing the core muscles and pressing your hand into the floor while slowly moving your right arm. Perform 6 to 10 repetitions, then switch sides.

Correct Your Form

Keep your hips and shoulders at the same level. Exhale as you reach your right hand under your left arm and inhale as you reach upward toward the ceiling.

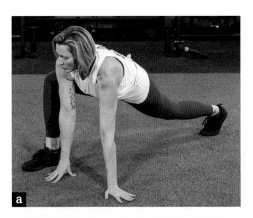

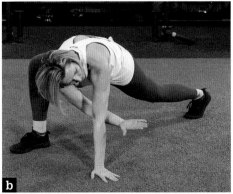

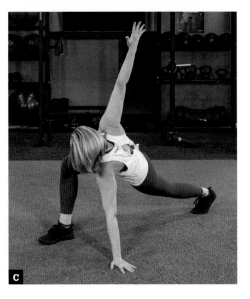

Bodyweight Workouts

Mobility workouts using your body weight are perfect for days when you are sore and feeling the effects of the workout from the day before. You want to do some exercise but not anything that will increase the feeling of soreness. These exercises feature just your body weight and gravity while you move through multiple planes of motion to get any residual soreness out of your system. The low-intensity muscle contractions will enhance circulation to help remove remaining metabolites that could cause soreness. To reduce any soreness you might be experiencing, complete at least two sets of each exercise move; if you want a little bit of a workout that won't overload your entire body, complete four sets of each exercise.

Exercise	Repetitions	Sets
Atomic frog hip openers	10-15 each side	2-4
Kneeling hip extension with thoracic rotation	8-12 each side	2-4
90-90 shin boxing	6-10 each side	2-4
Plank with rotation	6-10 each side	2-4
Reverse lunge with overhead reach	8-12 each side	2-4
Lateral lunge with thoracic rotation	8-12 each side	2-4
Transverse plane lunge with reach for the ground	8-12 each side	2-4

BODYWEIGHT MOBILITY

Atomic Frog Hip Openers

Benefits

When the hip muscles become too tight, they can change how the hips and knees function. This move looks a little awkward, but it helps improve mobility of the hips in the transverse plane, which can reduce stress on the joints above and below the hip.

Instructions

1. Start in a quadruped position with your wrists under your shoulders and your knees under your hips. Lower yourself to your elbows so they are directly under your shoulders while spreading your knees out wide so that the insides of your upper thighs are almost touching the floor (a).
2. Move your upper body diagonally toward your left shoulder while you pick up your right foot. Allow your hip to rotate so that your right foot moves away from the floor (b); this creates rotation at the hip joint, which helps improve mobility. Perform 10 to 15 repetitions with the right leg, then switch directions.

Correct Your Form

Use a stretch mat to reduce stress on your knees. Keep your spine long and straight as you perform the movements. Breathe deeply; exhale as you move forward into the stretch, and inhale as you shift backward between repetitions.

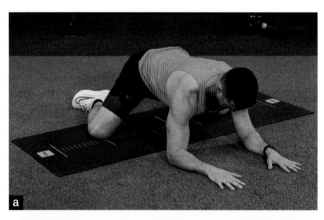

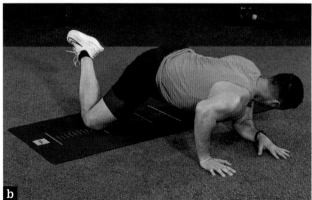

Kneeling Hip Extension
With Thoracic Rotation

Benefits

This exercise helps to activate and strengthen the glutes and quadriceps without putting downward compressive force on the lower back or knees. The exercise is great for using the muscles when they are still sore from a previous workout.

Instructions

1. Start in a kneeling position, with your knees on the ground and your tailbone resting on your heels. Keep your hands behind your ears so that your elbows are pointed directly to each side.

2. Extend your hips to come to a full kneeling position so that you are resting on your knees with your spine fully extended (a). Rotate and lean to your right as you keep your left hand behind your left ear (b). Pause briefly, then rotate your torso back to face straight ahead. Maintain the tall kneeling position as you complete 8 to 12 repetitions on one side, then switch sides.

Correct Your Form

Keep your spine long and fully extended during this movement. Breathe deeply with each repetition; inhale while moving into the tall kneeling position and exhale as you rotate and lean to the side.

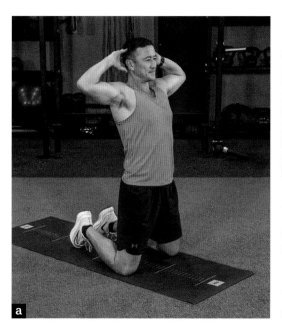

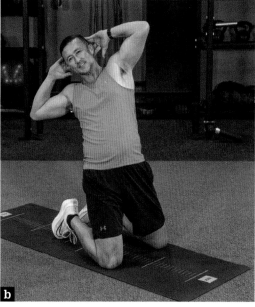

90-90 Shin Boxing

Benefits

This mobility exercise focuses on hip motion while seated, and although it can cause a little discomfort if the leg muscles are very sore, maintaining motion in the hips the day after a hard workout could keep adhesions from forming. In addition, this exercise helps to work on coordination and control of the hip and deep core muscles.

Instructions

1. Sit on the ground with your feet directly in front of you, your knees pointed toward the ceiling, your hands behind your body, and your spine in a tall and lengthened position (*a*).

2. Keep your spine tall as you drop both legs to the left side of your body (*b*). As the outside of your left thigh touches the floor, push your left thigh into the ground and hold it for 1 or 2 seconds before picking both knees up and dropping them to the right side of your body (*c*).

3. Focus on taking steady, deep breaths as you move your legs slowly from one side to the other. Complete 6 to 10 repetitions on each side.

Correct Your Form

Keep your chest raised and your spine lengthened to allow for optimal mobility in both hip joints.

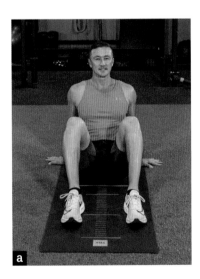
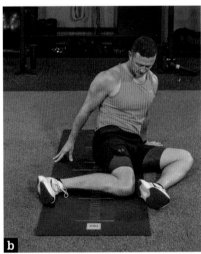
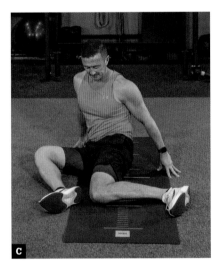

Plank With Rotation

Benefits

This move can help strengthen the upper-body muscles while enhancing circulation to remove metabolic by-products and deliver new nutrients to the tissues.

Instructions

1. Start in a high-plank position with your hands under your shoulders and your legs straight out behind you, squeezing your glutes and thighs to create extra stability (a).
2. Push your left hand into the ground and pick up your right hand as you rotate your trunk and upper body to face directly to your right (b) (both feet should be pointing to your right, your right arm should be reaching up toward the ceiling, and your gaze should focus up toward the ceiling). Pause for 1 or 2 seconds, then lower your right hand to return to the starting position and transition to the other side. Complete 6 to 10 repetitions on each side of your body.

Correct Your Form

Keep your spine long and your legs fully extended. Squeeze your legs together for stability and to make it easier to hold the position on one arm.

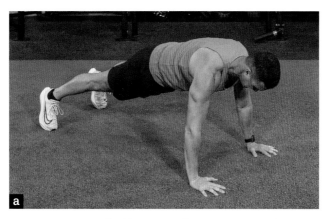

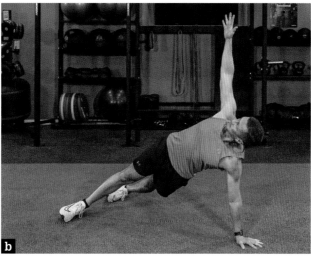

Reverse Lunge With Overhead Reach

Benefits

Increasing the range of motion of the muscles along the front of the hip improves hip mobility by reducing tightness and discomfort in the lower back. Stretching and lengthening the muscles of the upper back improves shoulder range of motion.

Instructions

1. Stand with both feet hip-width apart and your hands by your sides (a). Keep your left foot planted into the ground and keep your spine long and tall while stepping straight back with your right foot.

2. As your right foot reaches the ground, let your right knee bend to lower toward the ground as you sink into your left hip; as your body is lowering toward the ground, keep your spine long and reach overhead with both arms (b).

3. At the bottom of the lunge, pause and hold the stretch with both arms straight overhead for 2 to 4 seconds before pressing your left foot into the ground to pull yourself back to the starting position. Complete 8 to 12 repetitions, then switch legs.

Correct Your Form

Time the movement so that your arms are extended straight overhead while you are at the bottom of the lunge. Breathe deeply and focus on the exhale while reaching overhead with both arms. Focus on increasing your range of motion and control to improve mobility, as opposed to doing a certain number of repetitions.

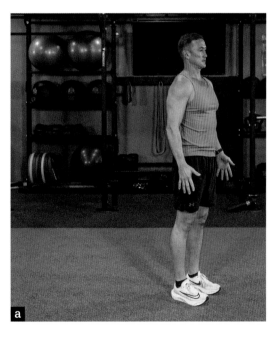
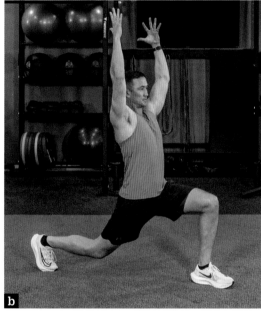

Lateral Lunge
With Thoracic Rotation

Benefits

Increasing the range of motion of the thoracic spine improves the mobility and strength of the hip muscles while increasing the strength of the core muscles responsible for rotating the trunk.

Instructions

1. Stand with your feet hip- to shoulder-width apart and hold both arms by your sides *(a)*. Step directly to your right; as your right foot touches the ground, make sure it is parallel to the left. Push the right hip back while keeping the left foot pressed into the ground; rotate to your right and raise both arms to chest height. Pull back with your right elbow while reaching across your body with your left arm *(b)*, which increases rotation of your thoracic spine. Turn your trunk as far as possible and, at the end of the range of motion, pause and keep your arms extended straight forward at chest height.

2. Rotate your trunk to face forward and push off with your right foot as you press your left foot into the floor to pull your body back to the starting position. Perform 8 to 12 repetitions to the right, then the same number of repetitions to the left.

Correct Your Form

Keep your feet parallel to one another during the lateral lunge; the left foot should be pointed straight ahead. As the right foot hits the ground, it should remain parallel to the left. Maintain length in your spine—the straighter the spine, the easier it will be to rotate (if you try to rotate while slouching, it could cause discomfort in your back). Keep your planted foot pressed into the floor; when stepping to your right, pressing your left foot into the floor will help improve mobility of the right hip.

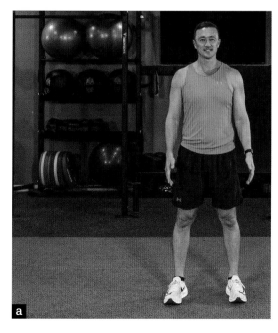
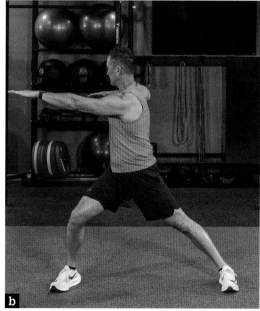

a

b

Transverse Plane Lunge
With Reach for the Ground

Benefits

This exercise improves the range of motion and mobility of the hips while strengthening the muscles of the inner and outer thigh; this helps reduce the risk of strains from overloading the fascia and elastic connective tissues.

Instructions

1. Stand with your feet hip- to shoulder-width apart (*a*). With your right foot, step back and away from your left (toward the 4 o'clock position on a clock dial); as you step to the right, placing weight into your right hip, keep your left foot pressed into the ground and squeeze your left thigh to help control stability of the knee.

2. As your right foot hits the ground, push the right hip back into a hinge position and bend forward to reach for your right foot with your left hand (*b*). (If you can't reach all the way to the ground, reach as low as possible; once your hip is in a flexed position, you can allow your spine to bend and round as you reach for the ground.)

3. After reaching for your foot, bring your trunk back to an upright position. Push off with your right foot and press your left foot into the ground as you bring both feet back to the starting position. Complete 8 to 12 repetitions on the right side before switching sides.

Correct Your Form

Keep your front foot (the left in the example above) pressed into the ground while stepping back with the moving foot (the right in the example above); push your front foot into the ground and use your inner thigh muscles to move you back to the starting position. Exhale as you reach toward your foot and inhale as you bring your trunk into an upright position.

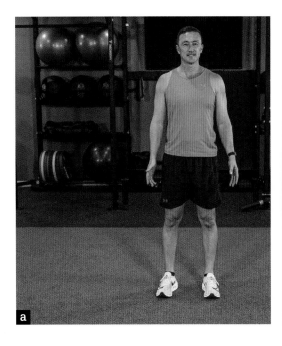
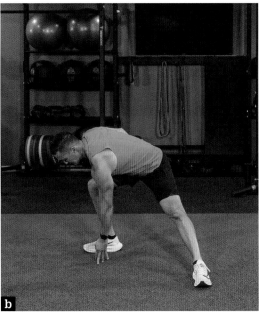

a

b

TRX® Suspension Trainer™ Workouts

Bodyweight strength training exercises can help improve mobility while enhancing muscular strength, and because they do not use any external resistance, they can be effective for promoting a complete return to homeostasis on those days when you are sore. Because there are only two points of contact (your feet on the ground and your hands on the handles of the straps, or vice versa), an important benefit of the TRX suspension trainer is that you are constantly engaging the core muscles that connect your hips to your pelvis and your spine to your shoulders during almost any exercise. Plus, because you can attach the TRX suspension trainer to a doorframe or a beam in the garage or take it outside to a favorite park, it is a great piece of equipment for home workouts. To reduce any soreness you might be experiencing, complete at least one set of each exercise move; if you want a little bit of a workout that won't overload your entire body, complete four sets of each exercise.

Exercise	Repetitions	Sets
Lateral bend and reach	8-12 each side	1-4
Hip flexor opener	8-12 each side	1-4
Rotating arms and feet	8-12 each side	1-4
Cossack squat with hip flossing	8-12 each side	1-4
Trunk rotation (push–pull)	8-12 each side	1-4
Rows	12-20	1-4
High plank with knee tuck	8-12	1-4
Gluteal bridge with hamstring curl	8-12	1-4

Lateral Bend and Reach

Benefits

The muscles along the sides of the body, especially the hip muscles responsible for stabilizing your knees, can become tight from being in a seated position for an extended period, which could restrict motion in the hip, thoracic spine, and shoulder joints. This and the following two exercises, the hip flexor opener and rotating arms and feet, are three moves that can help reduce tightness in and lengthen the muscles along the lateral and anterior portions of the body to achieve optimal posture, which is a requisite for effective mobility.

Instructions

1. Stand facing so the anchor point is to your right and your right foot is in front of your left. Turn your shoulders to your right to look at the anchor point while keeping your pelvis pointed forward. You should be far enough away so that there is tension on both straps when your arms are tucked into your ribs while holding on to the handles of the TRX (a).

2. Press your weight into your left hip as you stretch both arms straight and feel your spine lengthen (b). (This position increases the stretch into your back). Keep the tension on the straps the entire time. Hold your weight into your hips for approximately 2 to 3 seconds, then return to the starting position. Perform 8 to 12 repetitions on one side, then switch sides.

Correct Your Form

Breathe comfortably during the exercise. Inhale as you return to standing and exhale deeply as you laterally flex and move deeper into each range of motion.

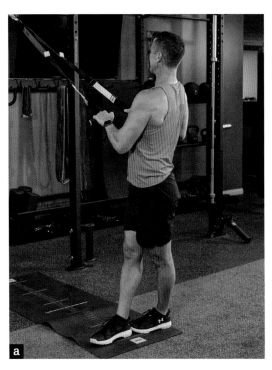
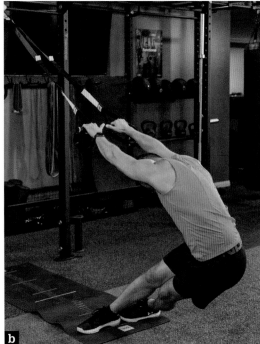

Hip Flexor Opener

Benefits

Your hips and shoulders work together when you are walking and running; this move uses the motion of your arms and shoulders to help reduce tension in the muscles that connect your upper body to your hips and legs. The result is improved mobility in your shoulders, upper back, and hips.

Instructions

1. Stand facing away from the anchor point with your feet approximately shoulder-width apart, keeping your left foot forward and your right foot back. You should be far enough away so that there is tension on both straps when your arms are extended straight overhead.

2. Stand with your feet shoulder-width apart and your right foot rotated to point toward your left *(a)*. Press both hands into the handles and straighten your right arm as much as possible while you rotate to your left and lower your left hand toward the floor *(b)*. Press your right hand into the air to keep the tension on the straps the entire time. Once you lower your left arm, slowly come back to the full upright, extended position to complete the repetition. Perform 8 to 12 repetitions on one side, then switch sides.

Correct Your Form

To increase the stretch on your hip flexors, contract the glutes of your rotating leg (the right in the example above) while lowering your opposite hand (the left in the example above). Relax your glutes once your left arm is back in the overhead position.

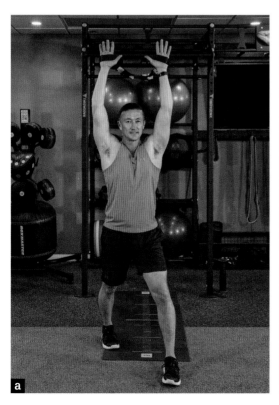

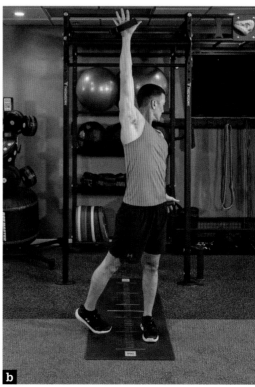

Rotating Arms and Feet

Benefits

The hips and thoracic spine are two of the most mobile segments of your body. Pressing into the TRX with your hands can keep your spine straight, allowing you to improve mobility of your hips and spine at the same time.

Instructions

1. Stand facing away from the anchor point with your feet shoulder-width apart. You should be far enough away so that there is tension on both straps when your arms are extended straight overhead (*a*).

2. Lower your left hand toward your left side while extending your right arm straight into the air and rotating your right foot to point toward your left (*b*); then, bring your left arm back overhead as you rotate your right foot to face straight ahead before dropping your right arm toward your right side and rotating your left foot to point toward your right (*c*). Your left hand and right foot should move together while your right hand and left foot move together as you rotate. Alternate from side to side and complete 8 to 12 repetitions on each side.

Correct Your Form

Keep your spine long and tall, and lean forward into the straps to create tension as you rotate from side to side. Breathe deeply and exhale comfortably as you perform the rotations and movements.

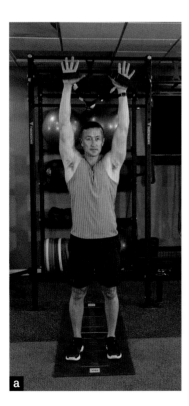
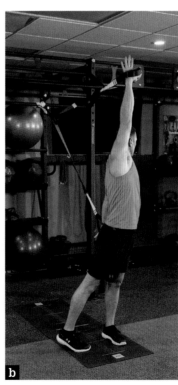
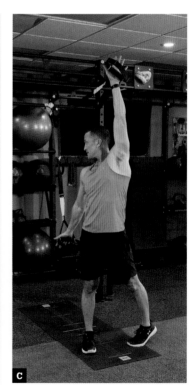

Cossack Squat With Hip Flossing

Benefits

When the hips become tight, they can place additional stress on the lower back and knees. This movement helps to increase hip mobility in all planes of motion so they maintain optimal function while lowering the risk of injury to the lower back.

Instructions

1. Stand facing the anchor point while holding the handles, with your feet wider than shoulder-width apart; you should be far enough away from the anchor point so that there is slight tension on the TRX straps (*a*).

2. Hold the handles as you sink your weight back into your right hip. Meanwhile, keep your left leg straight and allow your foot to rotate on your heel so that at the bottom of the move, all of your weight is in your right hip, with your left leg straight out to your side so that your toes are pointing toward the ceiling (*b*).

3. Holding the handles for support, stay in the low portion of the squat and push off with your right foot as you place your left foot flat on the ground and transition your weight from your right hip to your left hip (*c*).

4. Once all of your weight is back on your left leg, your right leg should be straight out to your right side. Press your left foot into the ground to return to a standing position. Once you return to standing, lower your weight back on your left hip before transitioning to the right at the bottom of the movement. Complete 8 to 12 repetitions on each leg.

Correct Your Form

Use the handles and straps to support your weight, especially at the bottom of the squat as you transition from one leg to the other. Focus on breathing deeply and exhaling as you complete each movement.

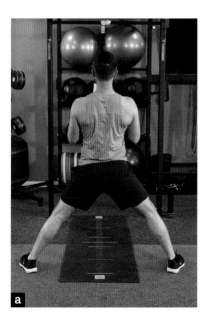 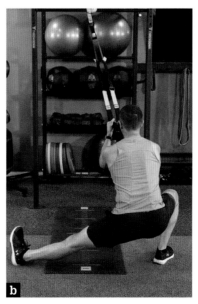 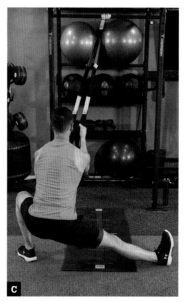

Trunk Rotation (Push–Pull)

Benefits

Combining two opposing movement patterns (pushing and pulling) creates rotation through the thoracic spine and hips, which can strengthen the hip and core muscles. In addition, the pulling motion with a single arm can strengthen the upper back muscles that help support good posture.

Instructions

1. Stand facing the anchor point of the TRX with your feet wider than shoulder-width apart. Holding one handle in each hand, lean back so the arms are fully extended (*a*).
2. Pull your left arm back over your left shoulder while rotating your trunk to your left as you press your right hand across your body. You can allow your right foot to rotate toward your left foot as you rotate over your left hip (*b*).
3. Pull your right hand back and rotate to your right, allowing your left foot to rotate to the right as you extend your right hand back over your right shoulder while reaching your left hand across your body. Throughout the movement, lean back to keep tension on the band while rotating from the hips. Complete 8 to 12 repetitions on each side.

Correct Your Form

Keep tension on the straps throughout the entire movement by leaning back. This also helps to activate the posterior muscles, allowing a greater range of motion in your shoulders and hips. When bringing your arm across your body, let your feet rotate in the same direction your hand is moving.

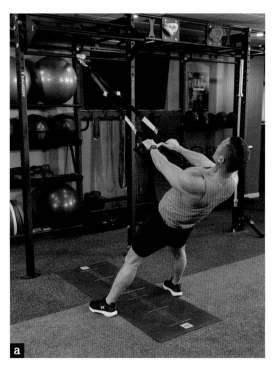
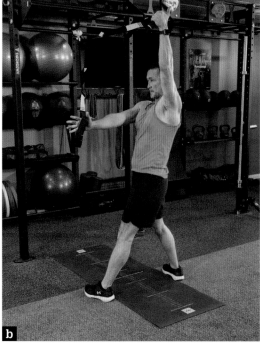

Rows

Benefits

This exercise uses the large latissimus dorsi, trapezius, and deltoid muscles of the upper back and shoulders. The movement of the arms helps to flush metabolites out of the muscle tissue, whereas keeping the hips and spine stable can help strengthen the deep core muscles.

Instructions

1. Stand facing the anchor point of the TRX suspension trainer, holding one handle in each hand.
2. Keep your heels on the ground and your legs straight as you lean back. When you are in position to start the exercise, keep your glutes squeezed and press your hips forward for optimal body control.
3. Start the move with your palms facing down toward the ground. As you pull your body toward the handles, rotate your wrists so that you finish with your palms facing each other. This rotation uses the forearm and biceps muscles, helping to improve their definition.
4. Keep your body straight as you slowly extend your arms to return to the starting position. Complete 12 to 20 repetitions.

Correct Your Form

The more vertical your body, the lower the resistance; the more horizontal your body, the greater the resistance. If you start fatiguing during the exercise, simply walk your feet back so that you are in a more vertical position. Grip the handles tightly in your hands, but think about pulling your elbows toward your ribs for optimal recruitment of your upper back muscles.

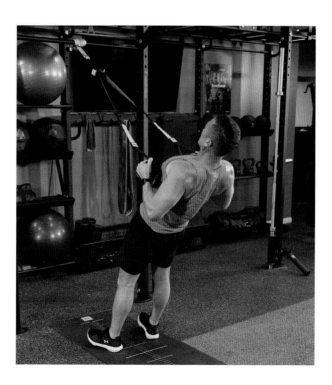

High Plank With Knee Tuck

Benefits

Placing the hands on the floor and the feet in the foot cradles (the fabric loops by the handles) creates a different challenge. There will be more stability in the shoulders, while the core muscles will work harder to reduce unwanted movement from the body. Pressing the hands into the floor while pushing the back up toward the ceiling can increase engagement of the core muscles.

Instructions

1. Place your feet in the foot cradles and press your hands into the floor under your shoulders, keeping your legs straight (*a*). (Pressing your hands down helps to activate the deep muscles that stabilize the spine.)
2. Lift your hips into the air as you bring your knees toward your chest (*b*). Pause, then slowly extend your legs out behind you. Complete 8 to 12 repetitions.

Correct Your Form

To increase stability while you are in the plank position, contract your thigh and gluteal muscles. Exhale as you bring your knees closer to your chest and inhale while extending your legs.

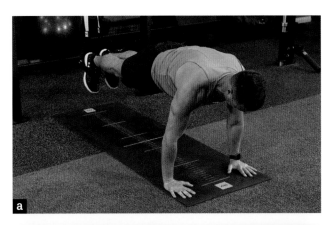

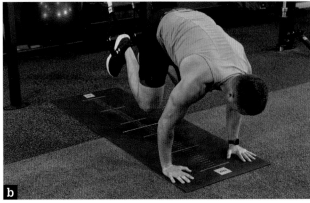

Gluteal Bridge With Hamstring Curl

Benefits

Lifting the hips off the ground and pulling the heels toward the tailbone can strengthen the glutes, hamstrings, adductors, and deep core muscles without the vertical compression created by a standing exercise, making this a great lower-body strength training exercise for days when the muscles are sore.

Instructions

1. Lie on your back and place your heels in the fabric cradles by the handles. Keep your legs straight and press your palms into the floor for support (*a*).
2. Squeeze your glutes to lift your tailbone off the ground while you pull your heels toward your glutes (*b*). Pause, then slowly extend your legs. Exhale as you bring your heels closer to your tailbone. Inhale as you extend and straighten your legs. Complete 8 to 12 repetitions.

Correct Your Form

Move your arms farther away from your sides and press them into the ground while your hips are in the air to increase stability. To increase the level of difficulty, bring your heels toward your tailbone quickly, then slowly extend and straighten your legs: 1 to 3 seconds in, 4 to 6 seconds out.

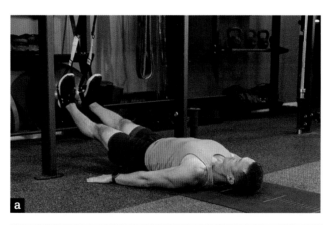

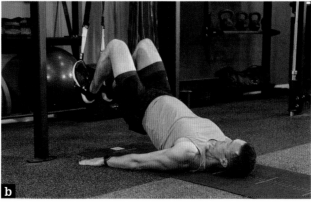

Cable Machine Workouts

The benefit of using a cable machine is being able to perform strength training from a standing position, which uses your muscles the way they are designed to function and helps improve overall intermuscular coordination. This low-intensity workout on a cable machine can provide the benefits of strength training while promoting the complete return to homeostasis; your muscles will be working to help burn calories and enhance circulation but not at a level of intensity that will create more fatigue. To reduce any soreness you might be experiencing, complete at least one set of each exercise move; if you want a little bit of a workout that won't overload your entire body, complete four sets of each exercise.

Exercise	Repetitions	Sets
Transverse lunge and pull	10-15 each side	1-4
Chop and rotation	10-15 each side	1-4
Standing crunches	12-20	1-4
One-leg balance with one-arm row	10-15 each side	1-4
One-arm chest press	10-15 each side	1-4
Squat to row	10-15	1-4
One-leg Romanian deadlift	10-15 each side	1-4

Transverse Lunge and Pull

Benefits

The many muscles of the core connect the shoulders to the hips. Exercises that use these two parts of the body at the same time can be effective for strengthening these muscles. This move uses the hips and shoulders in the transverse plane to develop a deeper connection between the two parts of the body and is an excellent way to strengthen the muscles while improving mobility of the hips and thoracic spine.

Instructions

1. Stand facing the cable pulley with your feet hip-width apart while holding the handle in your right hand (*a*).

2. Push your left foot into the ground as you step back with your right foot (place your right foot in approximately the 4 o'clock direction); as your right foot hits the ground, sink into your right hip and pull the handle all the way back to your chest while reaching your left arm straight in front of you (*b*). The combination of the pulling and pushing increases mobility of the thoracic spine.

3. Slowly step forward to return to the starting position. Use a weight that makes 10 to 15 repetitions challenging (the last repetition should be very hard). Complete 10 to 15 repetitions, then switch sides.

Correct Your Form

Think about creating push–pull forces with your legs; in the example above, push with your left foot; as your right foot touches the ground, press it down and pull your weight into your right hip while pulling back with your right arm (alternate sides).

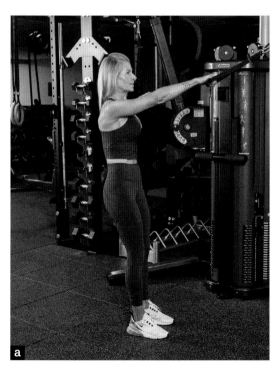

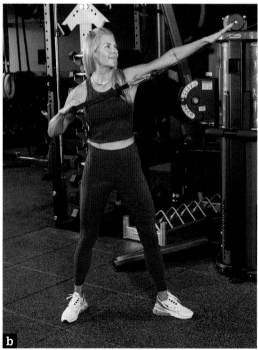

Chop and Rotation

Benefits

The rotation of the trunk combined with a lateral shift of the hips can help improve mobility of the hips and thoracic spine while strengthening the muscles responsible for controlling these parts of the body. The rotational movement of the hips and spine feels good the day after a hard running workout when these muscles are sore.

Instructions

1. Set the cable pulley above shoulder height and stand so the pulley is above the left shoulder. Hold the handle in both hands, with your right hand down first. Step back from the cable and move to your right so that your hands are directly in line with the cable pulley (*a*).

2. With the left side of your body closest to the pulley, shift your weight into your left hip; push your left foot into the ground as you rotate your hands in front of your body while shifting your weight into your right leg.

3. Keep both arms in front of your body as you rotate your torso, turning to face right; as you turn to your right, keep both feet planted on the ground. While shifting your weight into your right hip, turn your shoulders to the right. All your weight should be in your right hip (*b*). Slowly turn back to your left to return to the starting position.

4. Complete 10 to 15 repetitions on each side.

Correct Your Form

Keep your spine long and tall so that it can experience optimal mobility in the transverse plane. Pressing your plant leg (the left leg in the example above) into the ground will allow the other leg to rotate more efficiently.

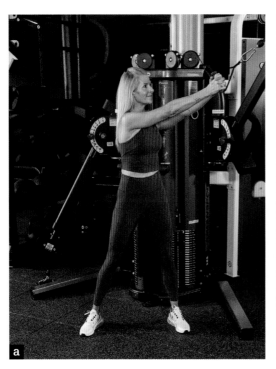
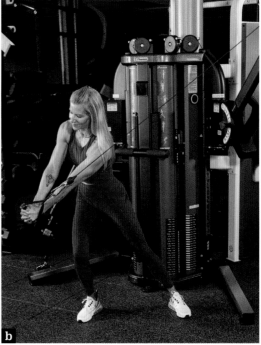

a
b

Standing Crunches

Benefits

The abdominal muscles help control movement between the rib cage, spine, and pelvis when walking. This exercise uses the rectus abdominis muscles the way they are designed to function, which can help improve their strength while enhancing circulation to promote recovery.

Instructions

1. Set the cable pulley above your head and stand facing away from it with your feet hip-width apart while keeping your pelvis level and your knees slightly bent. Hold the sides of the handles and keep the handle right over your head so that you are using your abdominal muscles to pull against the resistance (a).

2. Hold the handle with both hands while keeping your elbows tucked in to point toward the front of your body. To perform the movement, draw your belly button in toward your spine and shift your rib cage down toward the top of your pelvis (b). Focus on rolling your rib cage down against the pull of the resistance and slowly returning to the top. Perform 12 to 20 repetitions, then rest.

Correct Your Form

The abdominals attach from the front of your rib cage to the bottom of your pelvis, so the movement should focus on pulling these two body parts closer together, not bending or rounding forward from the spine. In fact, keep your spine long as you shift your rib cage downward toward your pelvis.

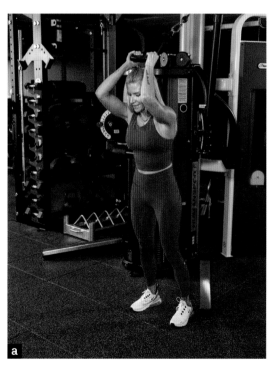
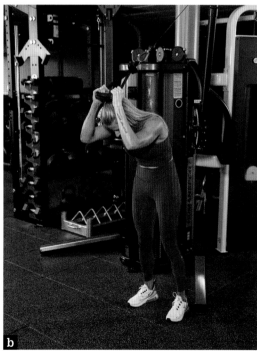

CABLE MOBILITY

One-Leg Balance With One-Arm Row

Benefits

Pulling from a single-leg balance requires using most of the deep core muscles that establish spinal stability as well as the muscles that control the hip to hold a balanced position. Balancing on the left leg while pulling with the right arm (and vice versa) strengthens the core muscles the way they actually function during activities like walking or running, making this an extremely effective move for strengthening muscles while promoting a rapid return to homeostasis.

Instructions

1. Set the cable pulley above head height. Kneel facing the pulley so that your left foot is forward and your right foot is behind your body. Extend your right arm and grip the handle with your right hand while keeping your left arm pulled back (a).

2. Press your left foot into the ground while squeezing your left glutes for stability. Slowly pull the cable back with your right arm while reaching your left hand forward (b). Pause at the end of the movement, and slowly step back while allowing both arms to return to the starting position. Complete 10 to 15 repetitions, then switch sides.

Correct Your Form

Having more tension on the cable helps you control your body. Start with the cable weight resting off of the stack, creating forward tension. When pulling back on the cable handle, think about pulling from your elbow (this is the attachment point for your upper back muscles and will help increase the fluidity of the movement).

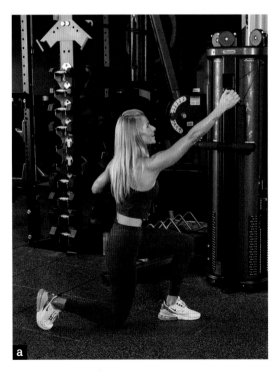

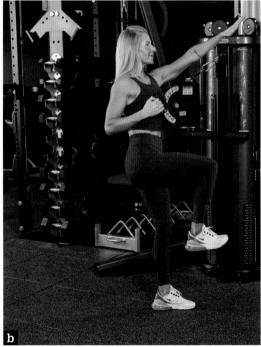

One-Arm Chest Press

Benefits

Pushing from one side of the body can help engage the deep muscles responsible for stabilizing the spine. In addition, chest presses from a standing position allow for a greater range of motion from the shoulder when compared with normal chest presses on a hard bench, which can help maintain or improve mobility of the shoulder joints after a hard workout.

Instructions

1. Place the pulley of the cable machine at approximately chest height; stand facing away from the anchor point and grip the handle tightly in your left hand so that the cable is directly on top of your forearm (your elbow should be directly in line with the pulley at the start of the movement).

2. Keep your feet shoulder-width apart and press both feet into the ground to enhance stability (*a*). Keep your pelvis level and press your feet into the ground to activate the muscles that stabilize your spine.

3. Keep your spine tall and press your left arm forward while pulling your right arm back. Pause at the end of the movement for 2 or 3 seconds (*b*), then slowly bring your arm back to the starting position. Perform 10 to 15 repetitions, then switch sides.

Correct Your Form

For optimal range of motion from your shoulder, keep your spine long and lift your chest as you press your arm forward. If the cable is moving over your shoulder or arm, make sure your elbow is directly in front of the cable pulley.

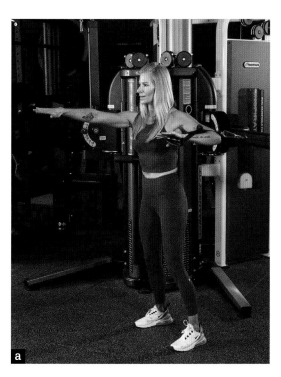

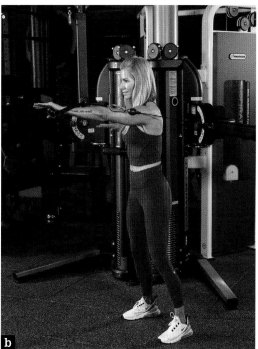

Squat to Row

Benefits

Pulling movements from a standing position can integrate both the large muscles of the upper back and the large muscles responsible for extending the hips and legs. Using more muscle mass can increase energy expenditure while improving strength.

Instructions

1. Set the cable pulley lower than waist height. Stand with your feet shoulder-width apart and facing the anchor point but far enough away so that there is tension on the cable. While you hold the handles in your hands, keep your feet hip-width apart and your spine tall and long.

2. Lift your chest, hold your arms straight in front of you, and push your hips back to lower yourself into a squat (*a*). At the bottom of the squat, continue to keep your arms extended and hold your spine long as you push your feet into the ground to return to the standing position. As you stand up, pull the handles toward your body while keeping your arms parallel to the floor and your elbows close to your sides. Your hands should reach the front of your body as you reach the standing position (*b*). Pause and slowly extend your arms as you drop down into the next squat. Complete 10 to 15 repetitions.

Correct Your Form

To increase stability, keep both feet pressed into the ground. Work on the timing so that your arms are moving forward as you lower yourself into the squat and moving back toward your body as you return to the standing position.

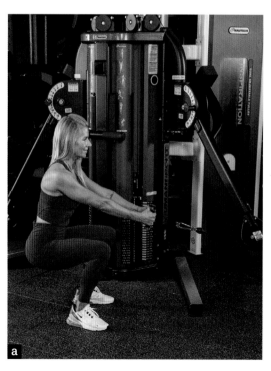
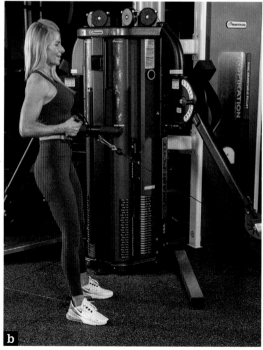

One-Leg Romanian Deadlift

Benefits

Exercising on one leg can improve balance and coordination while engaging the deep core muscles responsible for stabilizing the spine. This move engages the muscles of the inner and outer thigh at the same time, making it time efficient for both strength training and calorie burning. In addition, hinging at the hip while pressing the foot down into the ground can create a deep stretch of the hamstring and adductor muscles along the back of the thigh.

Instructions

1. Set the cable pulley in the lowest position. Stand facing the cable pulley, with your right foot directly under your hip, your right knee slightly bent, and your spine fully lengthened (your left leg should be next to your right, with the knee slightly bent). Hold the handle in your right hand *(a)*.

2. Push your hips backward as you begin to lift your left foot off the ground while pointing your left toes and straightening your leg. Keep your spine long as you point your left foot directly behind you.

3. Continue holding the handle in your right hand while hinging forward from your right hip to a comfortable distance *(b)*. Use your left leg to control the motion of your right hip, allowing the cable to help you maintain your balance.

4. To return to standing, push your right foot into the floor while pulling the bottom of your right pelvis down toward the back of your right leg while lowering the left leg down toward the floor. Keep a tight grip with your right hand. Complete 10 to 15 repetitions on each leg.

Correct Your Form

Control the forward hinging motion by straightening your left leg, squeezing your left thigh, and pointing your toes. Straightening your left leg will help you control the hinge on your right. Keep your spine long throughout the movement.

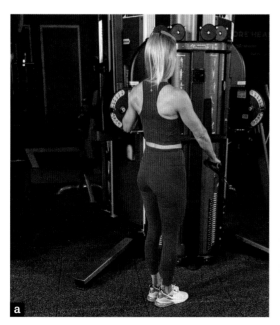
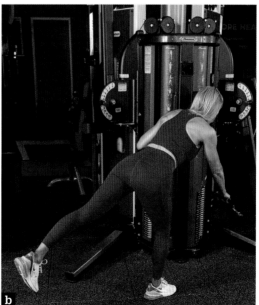

a

b

PART III

PLAN FOR RECOVERY

8

LONG-TERM PLANNING FOR RECOVERY

If you have been exercising for a number of years, it is likely that at some point, you hit a plateau where your body stopped responding to your workouts and your progress stalled. If the same exercises are performed with the same amount of weight, the same number of repetitions, or the same distance for an extended period, or if proper rest is not achieved between workouts, there is a high likelihood that your body will reach accommodation, the technical term for a plateau, where it will stop adapting to the exercises imposed on it.

Do you want to get stronger muscles with better definition? Resistance training to the point of fatigue can result in muscles becoming both stronger and more visually appealing, but it is important to adjust the amount of weight and number of repetitions so the muscles are challenged to work at different levels of intensity.

Do you want to improve your aerobic capacity and endurance? Running or cycling to exhaustion *can* help establish a higher level of fitness, but it does not need to be done every time you train.

Do you want to manage a healthy body weight? Exercising to the point of being breathless does help you burn a lot of calories, but it is not necessary for every workout.

No matter what your specific fitness goals are, changing the level of intensity of your exercise on a regular basis ensures that your muscular, metabolic, cardiorespiratory, neural, and endocrine systems will be challenged to perform at different levels of effort, which is the key to achieving long-term results. This does not mean skipping exercise the day after a really hard workout, when you are sore; it means you should plan to change the exercise intensity from workout to workout, which can be one of the most effective methods for avoiding overtraining and achieving the results you want.

Building Recovery Into Your Long-Term Workout Plans

As the previous chapter explained, exercising at a lower intensity can allow the body to repair itself the day after a really hard workout. Tools like foam rollers, mobility sticks, cryogenic chambers, saunas, compression clothing, percussion guns, and proper nutrition can be effective for promoting the return to homeostasis, but they can also be expensive. If you have the means, investing in these tools can help promote optimal recovery between workouts. However, two of the most effective methods of recovery cost nothing; they just need to be applied properly.

Rest is one of the most effective methods of recovery and can be achieved by applying the science of periodization to your workouts. In particular, improving the quality and quantity of your sleep can contribute almost immediately to your recovery and will be addressed in the following chapter. This chapter reveals a secret known by performance coaches who prepare elite athletes for competition: Achieving the greatest benefits from your workouts requires scheduling them so that your body has the chance to properly rest and refuel between high-intensity workouts. That's right—achieving optimal recovery is simply a matter of designing workout programs that allow for the necessary amount of rest between high-intensity workout sessions. Workouts that alternate between high intensity one day and lower intensity the next can provide the stimulus required to achieve your goals without the risk of overtraining.

Because exercise is a function of movement, and movement is a skill that must be developed over time, changing exercises with every workout is an ineffective and inefficient long-term strategy. To develop your skill or improve your conditioning for a specific activity, there must be some consistency in the exercises selected for your workouts, and they should be structured to become progressively more challenging as you work toward your goal, with periods of structured rest to allow your muscles to fully adapt and recover. This can be difficult to organize properly. Yes, you want some variety in your workouts to make them interesting, but here's an important fact about exercise: It doesn't matter what type you do, it just needs to be performed consistently, with the intensity and volume adjusted to make the desired changes to your body. Unfortunately, there is no way to guarantee specific results; what works best is keeping a consistent record of your workouts and how you feel during the recovery process, as mentioned previously. Making the effort to properly track and record how your training intensity makes you feel can help you to avoid overtraining while optimizing your results. There are two harsh realities when it comes to how the body adapts to exercise:

1. Changing workout programs too frequently does not allow the body to adapt to the work being performed, ultimately reducing the chance of experiencing the results you want.

2. Never changing the intensity or volume of a workout program means that your muscles and physiological systems will adapt to the exercises being performed, and your body will hit a plateau.

Designing Periodization Programs to Maximize Recovery

Following the same workout program for too long or changing your workouts too frequently are two common mistakes that keep you from achieving the results you want. After an initial adaptation phase of a few workouts, the more often your muscles perform the same exercise at the same level of intensity or run the same distance at the same pace, the less new stimulus they receive, meaning you will literally just be going through the motions. The same is true if you change workouts too frequently; the nervous and muscular systems respond to variation because it challenges them to work differently, but changing too often does not allow for the consistency necessary for long-term adaptations.

Periodization is the process of organizing an exercise program into phases of higher- and lower-intensity workouts and was developed specifically to maximize the recovery process for athletes preparing for a competition (Bompa and Buzzichelli 2015). An example of a periodized program for professional basketball players would be exercising to be in playing shape before training camps begin in late September and to achieve peak fitness when teams are making a push for the postseason playoffs in March and April. Once a National Basketball Association team has completed its season, the athletes will have a period of light activity not specific to basketball before beginning the conditioning program to prepare for the next season.

The science of periodization can provide a systematic way to change the volume and intensity of exercise. The basic exercise movements can be consistent to achieve muscular development, but the other variables of exercise-program design—intensity, repetitions, sets, rest interval, and tempo—can be manipulated to create challenging workouts. You're not an athlete, you say? Fair enough, but if the science of periodization works to help multimillion-dollar athletes perform their best on the field or court, then it can certainly help you get in the best shape possible. The greatest benefit of periodization is that it allows you to schedule workouts that apply an appropriate amount of exercise stress while managing fatigue and reducing the risk of overtraining (Hausswirth and Mujika 2013).

Adjusting Intensity and Volume

Periodization is a systematic method of designing exercise programs that create either metabolic fatigue, mechanical overload, or a combination of the two during workouts while allowing for an adequate amount of rest between individual training sessions in an effort to achieve desired adaptations. Periodization organizes the intensity and volume of exercise into periods of high, moderate, and low intensity to maximize recovery, and it features structured rest or lower-intensity workouts as a means of promoting adaptations to high-intensity workouts. Volume is the product of intensity (the amount of resistance used for strength training or the percentage of maximum heart rate achieved for metabolic conditioning), the number of repetitions performed and sets completed in each workout, and the number of workouts per week.

High-intensity exercise imposes the metabolic fatigue and mechanical overload that contributes to the desired changes to your body. A properly periodized program can alternate between phases of heavy weight with low repetitions (to create mechanical overload) and phases of light to moderate weight with repetitions to the point of fatigue (to impose metabolic fatigue).

Optimizing Recovery

During exercise, the body is experiencing metabolic or mechanical stress; however, it is the recovery period *after* exercise when your body repairs muscle proteins and replaces the glycogen (which stores carbohydrates for energy) used to fuel the workout. Structured, consistent changes to your workouts should adjust training complexity, intensity, and volume while allowing proper time to rest, rehydrate, repair, and recover. Most elite performance coaches use periodization to help their athletes reach peak fitness for competition, and you can use it to ensure that you achieve the necessary rest so you are properly recovered between workouts.

Periodization features two specific models of adjusting volume: linear and nonlinear. Each model offers benefits that make it more suitable for different goals. Let's look at the specifics of each.

Linear Periodization

In the linear periodization model, volume and intensity are inversely related; over the course of a training program, as the intensity of the workouts gradually increases, the volume (amount of exercise performed) should decrease. The goal is a gradual progression of exercise intensity that increases over a period of weeks or months with structured periods of rest, usually a week, to avoid the risk of overtraining and to allow adaptations to occur. Over the course of a linear periodization program, the most challenging workouts should occur before a specific date, such as the start of a competitive season or a single competition (Bompa and Buzzichelli 2015). Linear periodization starts with a specific date by which to achieve peak conditioning and then works backward to organize exercise programs into shorter lengths of time, based on occasional periods of active rest for optimal adaptation. In a linear periodization program, the segments of time can be organized into short-, intermediate-, and long-term time frames.

While linear periodization was created for athletes preparing for a specific event, like a running race, or the start of a competitive sport season, it can also be applied for nonathletes preparing for a nonsporting event like a wedding, anniversary, reunion, or vacation. The goal is to combine progressively challenging workouts with structured periods of rest, or lower-intensity activity, to properly prepare and condition for the event.

A well-designed program should achieve optimal conditioning three to seven days before the start of the competition, event, or season so that a brief period of rest will allow your physiological systems to completely return to homeostasis. The exact amount of rest will be determined by the duration and intensity of the training program in addition to the length of the competition or season. A short, one-day event does not require more than two or three days of rest, whereas you could benefit from five days of active rest featuring low-intensity physical activity before beginning a months-long competitive season. A few days of rest or low-intensity physical activity immediately before a competitive season can allow your body to recover and achieve a complete state of homeostasis so you start the season with a full tank of gas.

National Football League Preparatory Training

Here is an example of how professional American football players could use periodization to structure their yearly training calendar. Their competitive season runs from early September to early January (not including postseason games, which could include another four weeks through the middle of February), with about one game per week. The goal is to start training to be in football shape in March, at which time the focus is on developing a foundation of strength and mobility. As the year progresses toward the playing season, the athletes will increase the amount of position-specific conditioning and will perform three- to four-week periods of high-intensity training followed by a week of easy activity to allow for adaptation so they will have the necessary level of fitness before training camps begin in late July. Once the playing season starts, the athletes compete on Sunday, for the most part (there are scheduled games on Monday and Thursday nights, which disrupt the normal training and recovery schedule); thus, they do very light workouts on Saturdays and Mondays, saving the hardest workouts for Tuesdays, Wednesdays, and Thursdays with the primary purpose of reducing the risk of injury or loss of playing time due to injury and a secondary goal of enhancing their conditioning so they peak at the highest level of fitness when beginning to make a push for the postseason playoffs in late November. Once a professional football team has completed its season in January or February, the athletes will have a period of light activity not specific to football before beginning the conditioning program to prepare for the next season.

A National Football League (NFL) season lasts from early September through the following January. During the season, teams compete in one game during the week, most often on Sunday afternoon, and every game matters toward the end-of-year standings, which means there is a very structured schedule for both conditioning and the postexercise recovery period. The athletes need to prepare to be successful on the field, but they also need enough rest and active recovery time to allow the workouts to have an effect. The teams that figure out how to help their players recover after one Sunday so they can be fully and adequately prepared for the next have a distinct advantage over their competitors.

March: Start off-season conditioning program

April to June: Moderate- to high-intensity exercise to develop a foundation of fitness

July to August: Highest-intensity preseason conditioning to prepare for the competitive season

September to February: Competitive season; playing on Sundays and conditioning during the week, with active rest days on Saturdays and Mondays

If you have ever followed a program to prepare for a running race such as a marathon, where the mileage gradually increases each week and you are supposed to take three to five days of active rest before the event, that is an example of linear periodization. The greatest benefit of periodization is that it uses rest as a means of allowing for adaptation to the physically demanding stresses of exercise. Structured, consistent changes to an exercise program that adjust for training intensity allow you to maximize results while minimizing the risk of injury or becoming stuck on a plateau.

A linear program can be organized into periods of time for each training phase and should include occasional periods of active rest to allow for optimal adaptation to the exercise stimulus. In general, during the course of the training cycle, as the intensity of exercise gradually increases, the volume or number of repetitions performed should decrease. The periods of time are typically organized into the following cycles (Bompa and Buzzichelli 2015).

Macrocycle

A macrocycle is the overall time frame for a long-term program designed to achieve a specific, quantifiable performance goal with periods of active rest. A macrocycle may cover a period of months to years. The overall program should progress to a point of peak conditioning by a specific date or time. For example, members of a country's national team may be on a four-year training cycle to prepare and peak for the next Olympic Games. Another example would be an NFL athlete on a yearly macrocycle that begins in March and culminates with peak conditioning for a late December or January playoff run.

Mesocycle

Mesocycles are smaller units of time in which the training volume, intensity, and complexity are changed in pursuit of the overall objective of the program. Following the above example, a four-year Olympic macrocycle could be organized into eight six-month blocks of time, each of which has a specific training purpose or outcome leading up to the quadrennial competition. The mesocycles for an NFL player might be organized into periods of three to four weeks, followed by a week of low-intensity activity for active rest and adaptation.

Microcycle

A microcycle is the smallest unit of time for organizing a linear program. It can consist of individual workouts, days, or weeks. In a linear periodization program, each microcycle or mesocycle can become progressively more challenging based on training volume, intensity of the exercise load, or complexity of the movement patterns. A microcycle could also be a specific amount of planned time for optimal rest and recovery from the challenges of the workout program. An Olympic athlete might have four six-week microcycles in a six-month mesocycle.

Nonlinear Periodization

Nonlinear periodization uses more frequent variations in exercise intensity and volume to alternate workouts between higher and lower intensity within the same week (Bompa and Buzzichelli 2015). Changing the intensity and volume from one workout to the next can be one way to optimize recovery between workouts; the nonlinear model adjusts the variables of program design on either a week-to-week or a session-to-session basis. Nonlinear models apply varying levels of intensity to create desired changes while allowing for proper recovery between high-intensity workouts.

Nonlinear periodization may be ideally suited for general fitness goals, because it allows for frequent changes in intensity and volume that can be adjusted from one day to the next, whereas linear periodization applies a gradual accumulation of progressively challenging exercise over an extended period. Frequently changing the intensity of exercise can allow two or three high-intensity exercise sessions per week, and because you will have optimal rest between each one, you will be able to train your absolute hardest on those days.

In a nonlinear plan, Monday might be a high-intensity core strength training day with a kettlebell; Tuesday, a low-intensity metabolic conditioning day with a bodyweight circuit; Wednesday, a moderate-intensity mobility workout; Thursday, a high-intensity anaerobic interval workout with a kettlebell for metabolic conditioning; Friday, a rest day; Saturday, a high-intensity strength training day with dumbbells; and Sunday, a long walk followed by a low-intensity mobility workout.

The Power of Rest to Improve Fitness

Linear and nonlinear periodization models both recommend periods of rest every few weeks to allow the body to fully recover from and adapt to the stresses of the workout program. The primary purpose of a nonlinear program is to allow at least 48 hours between high-intensity training sessions for optimal protein resynthesis, muscle glycogen replenishment, and recovery from neuromuscular fatigue and for the immune system to perform its function of returning the body completely to homeostasis.

The nonlinear model applies varying levels of training stress throughout the course of the week, which can impose the metabolic demands required to make desired adaptations. If you like to exercise every day, nonlinear periodization allows you to change the intensity of training more frequently so you can keep your training intensity high for two or three sessions per week while allowing for lower-intensity workouts on the other days to reduce the risk of overtraining. This model also allows you to train for multiple events or recreational activities throughout a year, as opposed to a linear model of program design, which is structured to peak at a specific time.

The Secret to Gains

Whether you follow linear or nonlinear periodization, systematically changing the variables of your exercise-program design to adjust the intensity and volume can optimize your rest and recovery between workouts so you can achieve the gains you're working for. It can take your body approximately 6 to 12 weeks of consistent, progressively challenging exercise to experience adaptations; high-intensity workouts to stimulate change can be organized around low- to moderate-intensity workouts designed to support active recovery. It is well established that physical adaptations to exercise are the result of a progressively challenging program that gradually increases intensity to achieve a specific outcome (Bompa and Buzzichelli 2015). Again, this is where consistent record-keeping, both of workouts and the recovery process, can help to identify the optimal amount of rest between progressively challenging periods of training. Some athletes may require a full week of rest, whereas others can achieve optimal performance after only two or three days off. Recording and analyzing your data will help you identify the right amount of rest for your needs.

The Variables of Exercise-Program Design

Whether it's to add muscle size, increase strength, enhance power, or improve your aerobic capacity, every exercise program is created using the same basic variables: exercise selection, intensity, repetitions, tempo, rest interval, sets, and frequency of exercise sessions. How these variables are applied and the amount of rest you allow yourself between workouts will determine the results you get.

If you like to cook, then you understand that throwing a bunch of stuff in a pot and hoping it turns into something edible is not an effective way to prepare a meal. The first step of cooking is deciding exactly what to make along with choosing the ingredients required to make it. Similarly, the first step in designing an exercise program is determining the specific outcome you are trying to achieve and the types of exercise it will take to get there. The meal you want to cook will determine the specific ingredients and the best utensils, pots, and pans for the actual cooking. Likewise, your fitness goal will determine the best equipment to use, the specific exercises you do, and how often you do them.

To prepare a delicious meal, it is necessary to know how much of each ingredient to use, the order in which ingredients are added, the optimal temperature, and finally, the correct length of time in the oven or on the stove; the wrong application of any of these variables could drastically change a dish. Exercise is very much the same way. Performing exercises that are not relevant to your goal, using too much or too little resistance, or doing too many or too few repetitions could each drastically change the outcome of the workout. Just as the components of the type of food you want to cook will determine the process for preparing it, the variables of your exercise-program design will determine the exact ingredients you should use for a workout and how to organize them for the best results.

The variables of exercise-program design (table 8.1) can be organized based on what you want to achieve from an exercise program. Become stronger? Eliminate excess body fat? Prepare for a specific event or athletic performance? The variables can be adjusted to provide the appropriate mechanical or metabolic overload in a manner that allows for the optimal amount of recovery to meet your objectives.

Power Training

Although both strength and power can be enhanced by lifting weights, they are two very different outcomes. During a strength exercise, the muscle fibers shorten and lengthen to generate the mechanical forces required to move an external load. During a power exercise, the contractile element of muscle tissue shortens, placing a tension on the fascia and elastic connective tissues that surround individual muscle fibers. This is what generates the force to create explosive movement. Strength training increases the force produced by the contractile element, helping to enhance the amount of energy that can be stored and released by the elastic tissues. When the elastic tissues lengthen, they store mechanical energy, which is then released as the tissues shorten to return to their original size. Additional structural adaptations occur by increasing the amount of phosphagen and glycogen energy substrates and enzymes necessary for anaerobic metabolism that are stored in muscle cells. Power exercises can help increase the overall force output of muscle tissue while improving the resilience of elastic connective tissues and ligaments, helping to reduce the risk of injuries such as muscle strains.

TABLE 8.1 Variables of Exercise-Program Design

VARIABLE	DESCRIPTION	EXAMPLES
Exercise selection	Exercise selection is the choice of exercises performed during a workout. Your specific training goal determines the exercises needed to reach the outcome. If you're preparing for an endurance event, then it will be necessary to do a high volume of low- to moderate-intensity strength training exercises to help develop muscular endurance. If you're preparing for a sport requiring explosive power, then you should be following a workout that progresses from strength to power. For best results, exercises should be based on the foundational movement patterns: Squat Push Hinge Pull Lunge Rotate	Reverse lunge with overhead reach Gluteal bridges Lateral lunge with thoracic rotation One-arm chest press TRX rows
Intensity	When it comes to resistance training, intensity refers to the specific amount of weight or external resistance used. In general, heavier weights are used to increase muscle-force output (strength) and create mechanical overload, whereas lighter weights help improve the acceleration of force (power) and are used with more repetitions to create metabolic overload. When it comes to metabolic conditioning, intensity refers to the work rate, or the amount of effort expended to maintain a certain velocity. Intensity could be described by a percentage of the maximum heart rate, $\dot{V}O_2$max, ventilatory threshold, or RPE. The purpose of periodization is to manage the application of physical stress applied to the body by regularly adjusting the intensity of the exercises.	Percentage of 1RM 10RM 8RM 10-pound (4.5 kg) medicine ball Dumbbells, 80% 1RM Kettlebell, 8RM Percentage of maximum heart rate Percentage of $\dot{V}O_2$max VT_1 or VT_2 RPE
Repetitions	A repetition is a single, individual action of movement at a joint or series of joints that involves three phases of muscle action: muscle lengthening, a momentary pause for an isometric contraction, and muscle shortening. Repetitions and intensity have an inverse relationship; as the intensity increases, the number of repetitions able to be performed decreases. Heavier weights can induce mechanical overload in only a few repetitions, whereas lighter loads or bodyweight exercises can be used for a relatively high number of repetitions to create metabolic overload. Repetitions can also be performed for a specific amount of time. If this is the case, the goal is to perform as many as possible in the available period.	10 repetitions for a strength training exercise 40 seconds for a metabolic conditioning exercise
Sets	A set is the number of repetitions or length of time a specific exercise is performed before a rest interval to allow recovery. The exact number of sets in each workout is based on the available amount of time and the specific goals of your training program.	3 sets of a strength training exercise 2 sets of five 50-meter (55 yd) sprints
Tempo	Tempo is the speed of movement for an exercise. Time under tension (TUT), the length of time muscle fibers are under mechanical tension from a resistance training exercise, is another way to describe this variable. Along with intensity, TUT is critical for creating the desired stimulus of either mechanical or metabolic overload. A slower TUT can induce more mechanical overload; a faster tempo can create a greater metabolic response.	Moderate-paced tempo for a strength training exercise Explosive tempo for a power training exercise Slow tempo for a mobility exercise
Rest interval	A rest interval is the time between exercise sets. It allows replenishment of ATP stores in the involved muscles and recovery from neural fatigue. Proper rest intervals are essential for increasing muscular strength and allowing for optimal metabolic conditioning.	Resting for 30 seconds between individual exercises Resting for 90 seconds after completing a circuit of different exercises
Frequency	Frequency is the number of workouts or exercise sessions within a specific period, such as a week or month. Too many high-intensity workouts without proper recovery in between each workout could lead to an overtraining injury.	2 or 3 high-intensity workouts, 1 to 3 moderate-intensity workouts, and 1 or 2 low-intensity workouts a week

Abbreviations: ATP, adenosine triphosphate; RM, repetition maximum; RPE, rating of perceived exertion; $\dot{V}O_2$max, maximal aerobic capacity; VT_1, first ventilatory threshold (breathing rate begins to increase); VT_2, second ventilatory threshold (out of breath).

Power training increases the velocity of muscle motor unit activation, or the speed at which the central nervous system (CNS) communicates with muscle tissue. The major difference between strength and power training is that strength training requires the use of heavier weights, whereas power training relies on moving at a faster velocity. During high-intensity exercise, anaerobic metabolism fuels the muscle contractions while the explosive force production creates a mechanical overload on elastic connective tissues; this combination of metabolic fatigue and mechanical overload makes tissue-treatment strategies an important component of recovery immediately after a power-focused workout. Consistent use of a foam roller, massage stick, or percussion gun could help ensure rapid tissue repair so you are ready for the next workout.

Strength Training

Strength training is the process of using external resistance to create mechanical overload or metabolic fatigue to enhance the functional performance of muscles, improve physical appearance, or both. Strength training can greatly improve the magnitude of force output (strength), extend the duration that muscles can generate force (endurance), increase the velocity at which force can be produced (power), and enhance muscle size simultaneously. However, a different approach to exercise is required for each outcome. Strength training with heavy loads can impose mechanical overload to improve muscle-force output without necessarily increasing muscle size, whereas exercising with lighter loads to the point of metabolic fatigue could help to enhance muscle size without necessarily resulting in significant increases in strength.

Have you ever noticed how different athletes have completely different bodies? Bodybuilders develop large muscles with impressive levels of definition. Powerlifters generally have large muscles that are less defined but are capable of lifting an impressive amount of weight. Track and field athletes who compete in explosive events can achieve greater muscle mass and higher levels of definition compared with their teammates who compete in endurance events. Even athletes on the same American football team can have completely different body types based on the position they play. The differences in body types can be partly explained by how each individual athlete prepares for competition. The specific exercises performed to enhance athletic performance can also help to improve aesthetic appearance. Different types of strength training deliver specific outcomes; for example, training for power can increase force production for athletic performance, whereas training for strength with weights can help burn calories and change definition for an improved appearance.

Zatsiorsky and colleagues (2020) identify three specific methods of strength training, each imposing a different amount of metabolic fatigue or mechanical overload to disrupt homeostasis: the repeated-effort method, the maximal-effort method, and the dynamic-effort method.

Repeated-Effort Method

The repeated-effort method uses a nonmaximal load lifted repeatedly until a point of momentary muscle fatigue (the inability to perform another repetition). Achieving fatigue helps to ensure that all the involved motor units (and their attached fibers) are recruited while depleting all the available glycogen. Due to the high number of repetitions with a moderately heavy load, the repeated-effort method stimulates muscle growth and increases strength by creating both mechanical overload and metabolic fatigue. This method recruits type II, high-threshold motor units to sustain the necessary force production for a high volume of repetitions. Anaerobic type II muscle fibers create energy through anaerobic glycolysis, which produces metabolic by-products that could help promote muscle growth but that also must be addressed with appropriate recovery strategies. Research suggests that acidosis, the change in blood acidity due to an accumulation of blood lactate, is associated with an increase in growth hormone and insulin-like growth factor 1 to promote tissue repair during the recovery phase (Schoenfeld 2021). An example of the repeated-effort method is bodybuilding, a sport in which bodybuilders compete to see who has achieved the highest level of muscle mass and definition.

Tissue-treatment strategies such as foam rolling or using a massage stick can help promote circulation for a faster return to homeostasis, whereas proper nutrition can help refuel muscle cells so they have energy for the next hard workout.

Maximal-Effort Method

The maximal-effort method of strength training uses heavy resistance to increase the number of higher-threshold, type II motor units and attached muscle fibers that are activated in a specific muscle. Have you ever lifted, or tried to lift, a heavy weight and felt your muscles shaking? That was because the CNS was sending electrical signals to the motor units to generate the force needed to move the resistance. Maximal-effort training can improve both intramuscular coordination (the number of motor units functioning within a specific muscle) and intermuscular coordination (the ability of multiple muscles to time their firing rates to contract simultaneously). The primary stimulus of maximal-effort training is mechanical overload, which can greatly increase the force output of a muscle without adding too much size. An example of the maximal-effort method is powerlifting, a sport in which athletes compete to see who can lift the most weight in three lifts: the barbell deadlift, the barbell bench press, and the barbell squat.

Because the maximal-effort method imposes significant mechanical overload, optimal recovery strategies could include tissue treatment using a foam roller, percussion gun, or massage stick along with compression clothing and the use of a sauna. Proper nutrition with a focus on protein intake to help promote muscle repair is also essential, as is rest.

Dynamic-Effort Method

The dynamic-effort method is another approach to power training and applies nonmaximal loads while moving at the fastest velocity possible to increase the rate of force production of type II muscle fibers. Using a heavier mass to increase force output can slow acceleration but helps muscles develop the ability to generate greater force. Using a lighter mass can increase the rate of acceleration, resulting in greater power output. The dynamic-effort method causes the contractile element of muscle to hold an isometric contraction, which places tension on the fascia and elastic connective tissues. The dynamic-effort method could be the most effective means of increasing the rate of force development to produce the explosive power essential for many competitive sports. Examples of the dynamic-effort method include weightlifting, where athletes compete to see who can lift the most weight in explosive lifts such as the barbell snatch and the barbell clean-and-jerk, and the field sports of shot put, hammer toss, and discus, where athletes compete to see who can throw a weighted implement the farthest.

For all three strength training methods, when muscle cells metabolize fat or carbohydrates into adenosine triphosphate (ATP), they are using chemical energy for the contractions; muscles can also produce mechanical energy as the result of the stretch–shorten cycle (SSC) of muscle action. The lengthening (eccentric) phase of the SSC stores potential energy as a muscle lengthens, and the shortening (concentric) phase releases the energy as a muscle returns to resting length. Power exercises increase the velocity of force production by enhancing coordination between the contractile and elastic components of muscle to reduce the duration of the SSC. Minimizing the transition time between the lengthening and shortening phases of action can increase a muscle's power output but places a tremendous amount of physical stress on both the contractile element and elastic component of muscle tissue. Proper tissue-treatment strategies, such as using a foam roller, percussion gun, or massage stick immediately after a power workout and wearing compression clothing, could help improve circulation to remove metabolic by-products while reducing physical tension on the tissues.

Different methods of strength training explain why athletes may look so different—it has to do with the amount and type of muscle-force production. The purpose of bodybuilding is to achieve a high level of muscle mass and definition; therefore, these athletes apply the repeated-effort method to grow the largest, most defined muscles possible by increasing the ability to store both glycogen and water in muscle cells. Sports like weightlifting, rugby, American football, and soccer require explosive strength, speed, and agility for optimal success, making the dynamic-effort method the preferred strength training technique for optimum performance. The explosive movements of the dynamic-effort method enhance the neural efficiency of type II muscle fibers—their ability to contract as fast as possible. The result is well-defined but not overly large muscles. In the sport of powerlifting, athletes compete to lift as much weight as possible for a single repetition at a time, which is exactly what the maximal-effort method of training will achieve. Although each method has benefits, athletes who need explosive performance use primarily the dynamic-effort method of training to prepare for their specific sport; strength-based athletes use the maximal-effort method to achieve the greatest muscle-force output possible; and aesthetic competitors might prefer to use the repeated-effort method to stimulate optimal muscle growth.

Increasing Strength and Power Output

The CNS is a critical component of increasing both strength and power because it controls when and how motor units stimulate muscle fibers to contract. Muscle spindles are sensory receptors that identify changes in muscle length and communicate those changes to the CNS to produce the appropriate amount of muscle force. Muscle spindles lie parallel to individual muscle fibers and sense changes in muscle length as well as the velocity of the length change. When a muscle is rapidly lengthened, the muscle spindles are lengthened, and they respond by initiating a discharge of the alpha motor neurons that cause the involved muscle to contract (Verkoshansky and Siff 2009).

Muscle-force output is based not only on the size of the muscle or individual muscle fibers but on *intramuscular coordination*—the efficiency with which the CNS activates individual fibers within a particular muscle. This, in turn, is based on three separate components:

1. *Muscle fiber recruitment:* Rapid lengthening during the eccentric phase of the SSC stimulates muscle spindles to activate more muscle motor units within a specific muscle.

2. *Synchronization:* More motor units are activated simultaneously to increase the force output.

3. *Rate coding:* Motor units are activated by the CNS at a faster rate. In general, faster firing rates of muscle motor units lead to an increase in muscle power.

Intermuscular coordination, on the other hand, is the ability to activate many muscles at the same time to achieve maximal force output for a specific movement. Adaptations by the CNS are primarily responsible for increasing both intramuscular and intermuscular coordination, which ultimately enhances the rate of force production and total power output for a particular movement.

Table 8.2 identifies different strength outcomes and how to apply the variables of exercise-program design to achieve each one. The level of intensity and total training volume will determine the overall level of mechanical and/or metabolic overload and the amount of recovery necessary for optimal adaptation. Consistently measuring and recording your workouts and recovery process will allow you to identify which level of training intensity provides the optimal results for your goals. It may take more than one competitive season of record-keeping to identify the optimal ratio of training intensity to rest, but once you do, watch out—your gains will be unstoppable. Record those workouts.

TABLE 8.2 Intensity of Strength Training and Different Strength Outcomes

TYPE OF STRENGTH	PRIMARY METABOLIC PATHWAY	INTENSITY (MAXIMUM REPETITIONS)	TEMPO	REST INTERVAL, SECONDS	SETS	DURATION OF RECOVERY, HOURS*
Endurance	Aerobic	12-20 or more	Slow	30-60	1-4	About 24
Base strength	Aerobic and anaerobic glycolysis	6-12	Moderate to fast	30-180	2-5	24-48
Hypertrophy (muscle volume; repeated effort)	Aerobic and anaerobic glycolysis	10-15	Slow to moderate	30-90	3-6	24-48
Maximum strength (maximal effort)	Anaerobic glycolysis and ATP-PC	1-5	Fast	60-180	3-6	24-72
Power (dynamic effort)	Anaerobic glycolysis and ATP-PC	1-8	Explosive	30-180	3-6	24-72

Abbreviations: ATP, adenosine triphosphate; PC, phosphocreatine.

*The type of strength training performed, along with the level of intensity and amount of muscle mass activated during the workout, influence the duration of the recovery process.

Applying the Variables to Workouts

An exercise program does not need to be overly complicated to be effective, but it does require the optimal time for recovery between each workout. Simply changing one or two variables, such as the intensity, number of repetitions, or length of the rest interval, can significantly change the amount of metabolic fatigue or mechanical overload. When you're feeling fatigued from the previous day's workout, simple solutions can include lowering the intensity by using lighter weight (or only your own body weight), reducing the volume by doing fewer sets, or lengthening the rest interval to allow more time between each exercise. Each of these changes could support recovery by reducing the overall stress load on your body.

Because nonlinear periodization allows for frequent changes in intensity and volume when compared with linear periodization, it may be ideally suited for most health and fitness goals in the general population. For example, alternating high-intensity workouts that create mechanical overload with lower-intensity metabolic conditioning to improve aerobic capacity can allow muscles to recover from the stresses of strength training while working to improve aerobic capacity. For general fitness goals, you should strive to complete the following in a seven-day week: two or three high-intensity strength training workouts, two or three metabolic conditioning workouts that vary in intensity from low to high, and one or two mobility workouts that challenge your muscles to move in all planes of motion. Obviously, it is not possible to add an eighth day to the calendar, so this schedule allows for some adjustment and variability; in some weeks, you may be able to crush three or four hard workouts, while in other weeks, it might be tough to make the time for two or three moderate-intensity sweat sessions. Learning how to apply periodization correctly allows you to remain physically active and work hard to maintain a high level of physical preparedness while adjusting your workout schedule to the real-world needs of your life.

Planning a Week of Workouts

No matter what your specific training goals are, in order to perform your best, plan to do *no more* than three or four high-intensity workouts a week, allowing for at least one full day between workouts. On the day after a very hard workout, help promote the return to complete homeostasis by doing a low-intensity active recovery workout. Using the 1-to-10 rating of perceived exertion (RPE) scale as a guide for monitoring intensity allows you to create a weekly schedule that alternates between high-intensity workouts (9 or 10 out of 10 on the RPE scale), moderate-intensity workouts (7 or 8 out of 10), and low-intensity workouts (5 or 6 out of 10). You can engage in very low–intensity activity (1 to 4 out of 10) on active rest days. Creating a schedule that alternates in training intensity could ensure that when it's time to work hard, you are pushing yourself to your limits, and when it's time to let your body rest, the lower-intensity exercise can help refuel your muscle cells and repair the tissues damaged during exercise.

Also consider your evening activities when planning your workouts. For example, if your planned Friday night is watching TV at home, then you can do a hard workout that day, because you'll be getting a good night's sleep for optimal recovery that evening. However, if your nighttime plans include tickets to a show or a party that you know will go into the wee hours, then you're better off doing an easy workout that day and waiting until another day for a high-intensity session. This is because if you stay up later than your normal bedtime (and possibly consume more alcohol or marijuana than normal), you most likely won't get enough high-quality sleep to adequately recover from a hard workout.

One of the best routines you can form is to take time over the weekend to plan your schedule for the coming week. Identify the workouts you want to do and, if necessary, make plans with friends for your workouts (which could include group fitness classes). Taking time to schedule your workouts lets you plan the exact amount of physical activity your body needs for each day of the week.

Table 8.3 is a suggested guide for a great week of exercise. This schedule will give you an idea of how to incorporate variety and adjust for intensity while allow-

TABLE 8.3 Sample Weekly Schedule of Workouts

DAY	WORKOUT DESCRIPTION	RATING OF PERCEIVED EXERTION (RPE): 1 (EASY) TO 10 (HARD)
Sunday	Rest day Allow your body to completely recover from a hard week of training by limiting yourself to very low–intensity activity like a long walk or chores around the house. Think of this as filling your gas tank (of muscle cells) so you have the energy to completely crush your workouts during the upcoming week.	1-4
Monday	Muscle-force production (strength or power training to a point of fatigue) A force-production workout focuses on either strength or power training to achieve a specific goal; for best results, repetitions should be performed to a point of fatigue. Example: Barbell total-body circuit strength training	7-10
Tuesday	Low-intensity mobility workout to promote recovery As muscles are recovering from the high-intensity workout on the previous day, perform lower-intensity bodyweight exercises using the foundational movement patterns to improve mobility or enhance core strength. Example: A bodyweight mobility workout	4-6
Wednesday	Moderate- to high-intensity metabolic conditioning Typically referred to as cardio, the focus of a metabolic conditioning workout is to develop the ability to sustain energy production for a specific activity. Metabolic conditioning can help improve aerobic capacity, which is essential for a quicker return to homeostasis. Higher-intensity workouts that focus on anaerobic glycolysis as the energy pathway should be shorter, whereas lower-intensity workouts using aerobic energy sources can be longer. Example: A steady-state cycling workout at an RPE of 6-7	5-10
Thursday	Muscle-force production (strength or power training) Same as Monday	7-10
Friday	Low-intensity mobility workout to mitigate accumulated stress from the week Example: A yoga class that combines movement with breath work to promote active recovery after a hard workout	2-5
Saturday	Muscle-force production (strength or power training; the highest-intensity workout of the week) Follow the same workout as Monday and Thursday, but add an extra set for each exercise. If you have no plans in the evening, add a brief high-intensity interval training workout for additional metabolic conditioning.	7-10

ing time for recovery. Obviously, you should customize your schedule according to your needs and interests. This sample schedule would work well for someone with general fitness goals like maintaining a lean, muscular appearance and a healthy body weight. The strength training workouts feature total-body circuit training for optimal muscle activation and energy expenditure. For optimal rest between training sessions, alternate challenging, high-intensity workouts with less physically demanding, lower-intensity ones. For example, if a challenging barbell workout (a 9 out of 10 on the RPE scale) is done on Monday, then Tuesday's workout should be at an RPE of about 4 to 6; the lower intensity allows the body to perform some physical work while making a complete return to homeostasis.

Remember that sleep affects your ability to recover and exercise; therefore, your evening plans should guide your training intensity on the weekends. On days when you have evening plans and may be drinking alcohol, using cannabis, or getting to sleep later than normal, it is a good idea to perform low- to moderate-intensity exercise, because sleep will be disrupted and may not facilitate a complete return to homeostasis. However, on days when you have no social plans for the evening, you can exercise to the highest intensity possible, because you'll be able to get to bed a little earlier than normal for a complete night of recuperative sleep.

Planning a Year-Long Training Program

According to Haff and Triplett (2016), "Excessive loading, monotonous training and overly varied training can all result in occurrence of the exhaustion phase" (585), which is the first step in becoming overtrained. In other words, exhaustion is an accumulation of fatigue, which is the first stage of overtraining syndrome. A common mistake is exercising at a high intensity too often without taking time for proper rest and recovery between workouts. Applying the science of periodization allows you to use time and rest to optimize recovery. One benefit of scheduling an extended period of workouts is that you can plan for constant variation in intensity and volume, which could help ensure that you continue to experience results while avoiding a plateau or becoming overtrained.

You can break up the calendar year of 52 weeks into four distinct seasons, with each season being approximately 13 weeks long. One way to apply the linear model to your workouts is to change your workout programs when the seasons change; this would mean that as the calendar transitions through spring, summer, fall, and winter, you change your workouts to focus on different goals throughout the year. For example, during the winter, when you spend more time indoors, you might focus on developing maximal strength; then, during the late winter and early spring, you might transition to hypertrophy to develop a lean, muscular body for the warmer months. When summer is in full effect, the focus could be on power and explosive training so that you can enjoy your favorite outdoor activities. As cooler weather starts to return in the fall, you could emphasize mobility and bodyweight exercises to give your muscles a break from the activity over the summer; then it would be time to transition back to maximal strength training. Your entire program could be based around whether you want to achieve your peak conditioning for your favorite outdoor activities during the summer months or the winter months.

Case Study: Periodization

In previous seasons, Allison didn't give much thought to a structured training and race plan; she just entered a race and showed up on race day. However, now that she has moved into the master's category, Allison set out to plan this year's season so she could be competitive and try to earn a local age-category championship in either the 5K (3 mi) or 10K (6 mi). At some point, she wants to compete for both, but for this season, she has planned to focus on her more competitive distance as the season progresses.

Allison started the season with shorter 5K races before entering and competing in the 10K distance. The purpose of starting with 5K races was to build tempo and speed with the shorter distance, then start to compete in the longer 10K races as her aerobic capacity improved. The six-month race season started in early April and will culminate at the end of October, allowing for 12 competitions in an approximately 24-week series of races. Allison's goal for the season, her first in the master's age group, is to be competitive for the podium in one of the events. Rather than focusing on increasing her training volume, she has been using recovery strategies in an attempt to gain an edge over her competitors.

Her goal is to race two times per month, every other weekend, so that she will have plenty of time between events to fully rest, recover, and train. The first three races she entered were 5Ks; it wasn't until her fourth race (and second month of competing) that she moved up to the 10K distance. For the remaining four months of the season, her first race of each month will be a 5K and the second, a 10K; as the season begins to wind down, Allison will be able to make a decision about which distance to focus on for earning the annual title. From inadequate sleep to poor nutrition to a lack of consistent mobility training, focusing on the recovery component of her workout program and keeping a journal of her recovery practices has allowed Allison to identify a number of ways to improve her performance without having to do any additional exercise. Once a workout is over, Allison keeps track of which recovery techniques she uses and how they make her feel in the notes section of her smartphone. At the start of the season, Allison was anxious because she thought she wasn't training enough to be competitive. However, her results have been the opposite. Through her journaling, Allison is realizing that the time spent on foam rolling, meal preparation, and sitting in a sauna is indeed allowing her to improve her performance. Allison's journal entries are providing evidence that her gains are happening during the recovery phase after the training session, not during the workout itself, and this insight is allowing her to have her best running season since college.

Each 13-week season could be broken down into two 6-week subphases for more varied changes in intensity and volume. The result is that each season will have two 6-week phases of training, for a total of eight changes throughout the year; this can provide enough consistency for adaptation but enough change to maintain engagement.

Table 8.4 provides an example of a periodized program for general fitness. This program is designed around the goal to be outdoors and enjoy the warm weather during the summer, from July to September. The overall plan is to increase intensity in the warmer months to burn more calories and develop lean muscle mass, while reducing intensity during the cooler months to allow the body to completely recover from the stresses imposed during the summer. The colder months provide the opportunity for lower-intensity bodyweight workouts to challenge the body to move without the additional stresses of external loads. Transitioning to warmer weather means changing the volume and intensity to focus on increasing lean muscle mass and improving definition. Both hypertrophy and power training can be effective for providing the metabolic fatigue and mechanical overload required to change aesthetic appearance.

Keep in mind that this is just one example of how to structure a linear periodization program in different seasons of the year; there can be some variance in the dates to accommodate for life situations that can easily change plans. This is by no means the best or only way to organize a yearly training program, but it should give you a few ideas on how to use science to design successful workouts that could help you stay strong and avoid overtraining throughout the course of an entire year. No matter the specific training goal, the yearly program should change intensity on a regular basis to provide the opportunity for complete rest and recovery.

Rest is one of the most effective methods of recovery; it just needs to be done. That is exactly what periodization allows for—designing an exercise program based around rest. Yes, you can still do your high-intensity workouts. However, you might feel much stronger if you do only two or three hard workouts each week with optimal rest between each one, as opposed to trying to complete four or five hard workouts per week.

Exercise—more precisely, achieving optimal performance through exercise—is extremely important to you. You're not afraid of hard workouts; in fact, you thrive on them. Your fitness goals are important, so you want to be sure that you can perform your best when you are working out. In fact, you exercise so much that this book was written just for you, so that you can understand the role of rest in an exercise program. Yes, rest may literally be a four-letter word, but it is not a *bad* word. Your workouts are when you impose physical stress upon your muscles, but it's the time *after* the workout when the muscles are repairing and growing. Understanding more about your physiology and the role of the period after the workout can help you identify the best recovery strategies for your needs. As you plan your workouts, develop habits for your recovery so that you can be sure to achieve a rapid return to homeostasis after you are done sweating. Exercise. Refuel. Rehydrate. Repair your tissues. Rest. Train hard. Recover harder.

TABLE 8.4 Example of a Yearly Periodized Fitness Program

SEASON	PHASES	GOALS	DESCRIPTION
Winter	December 20 to January 28	Repeated effort—strength endurance	Exercise: Low-intensity bodyweight exercises and dumbbell strength training; total-body circuit training Intensity: 15RM-25RM Repetitions: 15-25 Rest interval: 45 seconds Sets: 4
	January 29 to March 18	Repeated effort—base strength	Exercise: Moderate-intensity barbell strength training; total-body workout Intensity: 8RM-10RM Repetitions: 8-10 Rest interval: 1 minute Sets: 4
Spring	March 20 to April 30	Repeated effort—base strength	Exercise: High-intensity barbell strength training; total-body workout Intensity: 5RM-8RM Repetitions: 5-8 Rest interval: 90 seconds Sets: 5
	May 1 to June 15	Repeated effort—hypertrophy	Exercise: Moderate-intensity dumbbell strength training; total-body workout Intensity: 12RM-15RM Repetitions: 12-15 Rest interval: 45 seconds Sets: 3
Summer	June 20 to July 31	Repeated effort—hypertrophy	Exercise: High-intensity dumbbell strength training; total-body workout Intensity: 10RM-12RM Repetitions: 10-12 Rest interval: 45 seconds Sets: 5
	August 1 to September 15	Dynamic effort—power training	Exercise: High-intensity explosive training with kettlebells and medicine balls; total-body workout Intensity: 5RM-8RM Repetitions: 5-8 Rest interval: 1 minute Sets: 3
Fall	September 20 to October 31	Repeated effort—strength endurance	Exercise: Low-intensity bodyweight mobility and strength training exercises; total-body workout Intensity: 15RM-25RM Repetitions: 15-25 Rest interval: 45 seconds Sets: 3
	November 1 to December 15	Repeated effort—base strength	Exercise: Moderate-intensity barbell strength training; total-body workout Intensity: 8RM-10RM Repetitions: 8-10 Rest interval: 1 minute Sets: 3

Abbreviation: RM, repetition maximum.

9

HEALTHY HABITS TO PROMOTE RECOVERY

This exercise book is unique in that it is not about exercise itself but rather what to do after you exercise to ensure that your workouts have the greatest effect possible. The focus of the previous chapters was on how to optimize postworkout recovery—specifically, what can be done on the day of and the day after high-intensity workouts to facilitate a rapid return to homeostasis. In addition, you learned how to schedule workouts that alternate between higher-intensity training to stimulate adaptations and lower-intensity exercise to allow those adaptations to occur. You have no doubt made exercise a consistent habit; it is now time to do the same with your recovery practice. Yes, in the hustle and bustle of modern life, it can be difficult to adopt new habits, but do not wait until you feel fatigued or start experiencing pain to make time for postworkout recovery. Applying recovery strategies as a regular habit can help you optimize your fitness levels while reducing the risk of developing a debilitating injury.

This chapter will focus on the long-term healthy habits that could help to reduce the overall stress load in your body so you can experience optimal recovery after high-intensity workouts. The key ingredients to recovery are refueling, rehydration, rest, and (tissue) repair, but because those are best applied once the workout is over, the question becomes what habits can you establish and what can you be doing on an ongoing basis to improve your body's ability to return to homeostasis after a hard workout?

Develop a Recovery Plan for Your Training Program

As you begin to develop your recovery plan and establish effective postworkout habits, keep the following principles in mind.

1. Accept the fact that it is not a good idea to perform high-intensity exercise for every workout. Instead, periodize the intensity of your workouts so you can achieve peak condition when you want it. At the very least, plan for at least one to two weeks of low-intensity activity or active rest every year to allow your body periods of complete rest. This could happen during a busy

time at work, such as preparing the annual budget or attending a conference; your body can achieve a complete return to homeostasis while you are focused on work activities. For example, if you know that the hardest part of your annual budget planning is the last week of September, plan your workouts for that week to be minimal so that your body can rest. Then, once your budget is done and approved, you can return to your normal work and training schedule. If you know you will be busy at work, make that time benefit your fitness by planning a structured rest from your workouts.

2. Stay hydrated and drink plenty of water throughout the day so that your blood has the ability to transport vital oxygen and nutrients to the working muscles. If you start to get dehydrated, it will have an immediate effect on performance; maintain optimal hydration to achieve optimal performance.

3. Pay attention to your nutrition. This does *not* mean dieting or cutting calories for weight loss. In fact, it's quite the opposite—fat and carbohydrates provide energy for physical activity, and fat is also essential for many hormones that control cellular functions. If your fitness goals require high-intensity exercise, you should know the basic role that nutrition plays in providing fuel for your activity. The nutrition information in this chapter will address the roles of each macronutrient along with the recommended daily intake levels of protein, because it supports muscle repair, and carbohydrate, because it supplies energy, for active or extremely active individuals. The point is to help you understand how much energy you need to fuel your workouts, as well as strategies for using nutrition to support the recovery process once a workout is over.

4. Sleep. This is one of the most important components of recovery and is something you already do, but just may not do enough. Sleep is the time when your body repairs tissues and replaces energy stores, so it should play an essential role in your overall fitness program.

5. Understand the role of meditation as an essential aspect of recovery. The brain is very involved in exercise, and meditation can be an effective way to strengthen it for the rigors of high-intensity training as well as help it to recover once exercise is finished.

Your Metabolism

Energy is neither created nor destroyed; it is transferred from one state to another. Metabolism refers to the chemical reactions required for converting the food consumed in your diet into the energy needed to support the body's normal physiological functions. The macronutrients you eat—protein, fat, and carbohydrates—support tissue repair, facilitate the production of hormones, or are metabolized into adenosine triphosphate (ATP), which is used immediately in the release of kinetic energy or stored as potential energy in the form of glycogen in muscle cells (or fatty acids in adipose tissue). Fats and carbohydrates are the main sources of ATP. The primary purpose of protein is to repair damaged tissues, although, as mentioned previously, it can also be metabolized into ATP to conserve glucose through the process of gluconeogenesis (Kenney, Wilmore, and Costill 2022).

Establishing Habits

When it comes to establishing a habit, focusing on the positive aspects of the behavior can make it a more pleasurable experience. Think of recovery as a calorie-free, postworkout treat—a reward for completing a grueling workout. A postworkout recovery strategy, like using a percussion gun to reduce tightness in sore muscles, becomes a reward for a job well done during the workout. The brain responds to pleasurable experiences by increasing levels of the neurotransmitters dopamine and serotonin; having a positive mindset toward recovery and learning how to enjoy the different techniques could help to elevate levels of these transmitters so that the time you spend on your recovery practice becomes a positive and rewarding experience. Here are a few suggestions for how to establish recovery practices as a consistent habit.

Add mobility and active recovery workouts to your schedule. And do them. If you live by your calendar, it can feel overwhelming when your schedule takes over your life, and it can be easy to skip a workout that doesn't excite you or make you feel like you're burning a ton of calories. However, mobility and active recovery workouts are an important component of the recovery process and can help you remain injury-free. Adding a mobility or active recovery workout the day after a high-intensity exercise session can give you the perception of being active while allowing the time for your body to completely return to homeostasis.

Keep a training journal, or, at the very least, a recovery journal. This doesn't need to be extensive and could easily be done in the notes section of your smartphone; all that is required is to record which techniques you used, for how long, and how they made you feel immediately after the workout as well as the next morning. One recovery technique may provide immediate, short-term relief that disappears by the morning, while another may not provide any noticeable change. Writing down how each recovery technique makes you feel could help you identify which are the most effective for reducing your overall stress levels.

Make your workout partner your recovery partner. Establishing a habit by yourself can be tough. However, having a friend along for the journey could help make the process a little easier. If you have workout partners, speak with them about the need to add certain recovery protocols to your routine. It could be as simple as making a few minutes for myofascial release using a foam roller or percussion gun or as extensive as going to a studio that offers cryotherapy and an infrared sauna. Just like working out with someone can make it more enjoyable, taking a trip to −300 degrees in a cryo chamber can be a little easier when a friend is there for support. Plus, the two of you can hold one another accountable for making the time for recovery treatment after each high-intensity workout. Committing to practicing recovery with your workout partner will benefit both of you on the way to establishing it as a regular habit. As with any component of an exercise program, it's only when the practice becomes a consistent habit that you will experience lasting and long-term results from your efforts.

Food provides energy, and high-intensity exercise requires an appropriate number of calories to fuel your workouts. Ideally, the amount of energy you consume is adequate to fuel the physical activity you perform. Not consuming enough energy results in a calorie deficit, requiring reserves of stored energy to be used to fuel activity. This could result in weight loss and keep you from reaching a performance goal. On the other hand, consuming more energy than is needed may result in a surplus of energy and weight gain in the form of fat. Identifying your specific caloric needs based on your activity level will ensure that you are properly fueled for your workouts and are taking in appropriate nutrition to support the recovery process.

Your metabolism is always working to burn energy. During periods of activity, such as moderate- to high-intensity exercise or frantically cleaning before your mother-in-law comes for a visit, your body will burn more calories than while at rest. (A calorie is a unit of energy equal to the energy required to heat one liter [34 oz] of water by one degree centigrade.) How we burn energy or expend calories, technically known as our total daily energy expenditure (TDEE), can be organized into the following categories (Kenney, Wilmore, and Costill 2022).

Resting Metabolic Rate

The resting metabolic rate (RMR, also known as the basal metabolic rate) accounts for approximately 60 to 75 percent of the TDEE. The RMR is the amount of energy used to support the functions of the body's organs and physiological systems while in a state of rest. It is the daily energy output required just to maintain homeostasis and does not include the energy needed for physical activity. The combined energy expenditure of the heart, lungs, kidneys, skeletal muscle, brain, and liver is approximately 80 percent of the RMR; the three organs most responsible for burning calories at rest are the liver, brain, and skeletal muscle, which account for 27, 19, and 18 percent of the RMR, respectively. The brain uses about 20 percent of the RMR to fuel the ability to collect and process information, which explains why you don't think as clearly when you're hungry. Muscle tissue itself is metabolically active and can burn between 4.5 and 7.0 calories per pound (9.9 to 15.4 calories per kg) each day, which means that adding 5 pounds (2.3 kg) of lean muscle should increase your RMR anywhere from 22.5 to 35 calories per day. When exercise adds lean muscle mass, it is time to increase caloric intake to make sure those muscles are properly fueled.

Thermic Effect of Food

The thermic effect of food accounts for up to 10 percent of the TDEE. This accounts for the energy required to convert the food you eat into more energy, or to move it to a location to be stored (as fat) for use at a later time.

Thermic Effect of Physical Activity

The thermic effect of physical activity accounts for 15 to 30 percent of the TDEE. This proportion includes excess postexercise oxygen consumption and nonexercise activity thermogenesis (NEAT). Exercise is physical activity for a specific purpose; NEAT refers to the nonexercise physical activities you perform throughout your day, such as going up a flight of stairs or walking to the store. When calculating your daily caloric intake, it is necessary to factor in both exercise and NEAT so that you can be sure you are consuming an appropriate amount of fuel.

Understanding the components of your metabolism can help to identify the ideal number of calories to support your exercise and physical activity. A nutrition plan should be personalized for your specific energy needs while factoring in your activity level, age, gender, and training. Your specific activity levels determine your daily energy needs. On days when your workouts are programmed to be high intensity, eating more can help fuel those workouts or replace the fuel after the workouts are over. When you're not training as hard, you can adjust the total intake to what your body needs.

Fueling Your Performance

This section provides general information about the hormones that support the digestive process as well as the role that macronutrients—fat, protein, and carbohydrates—play in supporting your workouts. Think of your body as a high-performance sports car. Are you going to use the cheapest gas, or will you pay extra for the high-octane, premium fuel recommended by your mechanic? Nutrition is the fuel for your performance. We will look at *how much* to eat to provide fuel for your body's needs during a workout and promote tissue repair and energy replacement after the workout; *what* to eat is completely a personal preference and will not be addressed. Therefore, it is highly recommended to work with a registered dietitian-nutritionist (RDN) to create a nutrition plan for your specific needs; go to the website of the Academy of Nutrition and Dietetics to find a licensed RDN in your area: www.eatrightpro.org.

Hormones and Metabolism

Nutrient intake, or food consumed, stimulates the endocrine system to produce certain hormones that metabolize macronutrients into the ATP that fuels all cellular activity, including muscle contractions. Hormones are chemicals produced by glands, and they control how cells and tissues function. A hormone can only react with specific binding receptors in cells; peptide hormones, for example, interact with receptors on the cell membrane, whereas steroid hormones interact with receptors on the nucleus of a cell. Hormones function to either stimulate or inhibit reactions within specific cells that contain the appropriate receptors, and many different hormones support metabolism to ensure energy availability. Consuming the necessary amount of energy to fuel your workouts not only ensures that optimal amounts of energy are available for your needs but can support optimal endocrine function so that all of your systems perform correctly while you are working hard.

Hunger Hormones: Ghrelin and Leptin

The hormones ghrelin and leptin control hunger and satiety, respectively. Ghrelin is produced by the stomach and stimulates feelings of hunger by creating a direct connection between the gut, where food is digested, and the brain, where the hormone crosses the blood–brain barrier to stimulate the lateral hypothalamus and create the signal for hunger. Leptin is produced by fat cells in adipose tissue to suppress hunger and stimulate energy expenditure. Research indicates that people with obesity have higher levels of ghrelin and lower levels of leptin, which could result in the tendency to consume too many calories at mealtime (Meier and Gressner 2004). It is also worth noting that inadequate sleep could result in elevated levels of ghrelin and lower amounts of leptin. Improving the quality and quantity of your sleep could help to establish the optimal levels of ghrelin and leptin needed to control hunger, which is a key component for maintaining a healthy body weight.

Hormones That Regulate Blood Glucose: Glucagon and Insulin

To help ensure that energy is always available or stored where it can be accessed when needed, the pancreas produces glucagon, which increases the amount of glucose available in blood or insulin to promote the storage of glucose in tissues (Kenney, Wilmore, and Costill 2022). Glucagon is released in response to low levels of blood sugar to stimulate the release of free fatty acids (FFAs) from adipose tissue and to increase blood glucose levels, both of which are important sources of the ATP used during exercise. When more glucose is needed during exercise, glucagon can release additional glycogen stored in the liver, which is then converted to glucose before being metabolized to ATP. When food is consumed and is in the process of being digested, glucose is released into the bloodstream. In response, the pancreas releases insulin to promote the storage and absorption of

Case Study: Calculating Daily Energy Needs

Energy is required to fuel all activities in the human body, from digestion and absorption of macronutrients to muscular contraction for movement. Physical activity, especially high-intensity exercise, requires a tremendous amount of energy, and your dietary intake should provide the energy needed to fuel your workouts. Identifying your RMR and adjusting it for your daily activity levels can help you identify the appropriate number of calories to consume to crush your workouts and optimize your recovery (table 9.1).

The Mifflin–St. Jeor equation (Mifflin et al. 1990) uses your body weight (BW), height (HT), and age to help you determine your RMR so that you can plan daily caloric intake to fuel your body and support postexercise recovery.

Mifflin–St. Jeor Equation for Estimating RMR (Calories per Day)

Women: RMR = (9.99 × BW [kg]) + (6.25 × HT [cm]) – (4.92 × age) – 161

Men: RMR = (9.99 × BW [kg]) + (6.25 × HT [cm]) – (4.92 × age) + 5

Table 9.1   An Individual's Physical Activity Influences the Resting Metabolic Rate

CATEGORY	PHYSICAL ACTIVITY	ACTIVITY SCORE
Sedentary	Less than 30 minutes of physical activity per day	1.2
Lightly active	Light exercise or physical activity 1-3 days per week	1.375
Moderately active	Moderate exercise 3-5 days per week	1.55
Very active	Hard exercise 6-7 days per week	1.725
Extremely active	Very hard exercise (or physical labor) 6-7 days per week	1.9

Allison is a 145-pound (66 kg), 35-year-old woman who is five feet, six inches (168 cm) tall and exercises every day of the week during the running season. Her daily caloric energy needs would be calculated as follows:

glucose by the cells to reduce blood glucose levels. Glucose is stored as glycogen in liver and muscle cells, and excess glucose can be stored in the fat cells of adipose tissue. At the start of exercise, the sympathetic nervous system suppresses the release of insulin so that glucose can be more readily available to fuel muscle activity (Kenney, Wilmore, and Costill 2022).

Energy Hormones: Cortisol, Epinephrine, and Norepinephrine

Cortisol is a steroid hormone produced by the adrenal gland in response to stress, low blood sugar, and exercise. Cortisol supports energy metabolism during exercise by facilitating the breakdown of triglycerides and carbohydrates to create the glucose necessary to help fuel exercise. It can also inhibit protein synthesis and reduce the inflammation that is essential for postexercise tissue repair (Kenney, Wilmore, and Costill 2022). To preserve blood glucose levels or when glucose is not readily available, cortisol can convert protein to glucose via a process called gluconeogenesis.

$$(9.99 \times 66) + (6.25 \times 168) - (4.92 \times 35) - 161$$

$$659 + 1{,}050 - 172 - 161 = 1{,}376$$

Allison requires 1,376 calories of energy to maintain homeostasis *before* any physical activity. Because she is very active, the total number of calories necessary to fuel her TDEE on the days she performs high-intensity exercise is $1{,}376 \times 1.725 = 2{,}374$.

On the days when she does lower-intensity exercise, she should adjust her caloric intake to reflect the lower activity level, so 1,376 should be multiplied by 1.375, which results in 1,892 calories—a difference of almost 500 calories per day. On high-intensity workout days, having a 500-calorie snack or meal immediately after the workout can supply the energy needed to replace what was used during exercise.

Throughout the season, Allison has worked with her RDN to develop a meal-planning schedule that is relatively consistent with her periodization schedule; on high-intensity workout and race days, more fuel is needed for the workout or to support postexercise recovery. On days when workouts are focused on active recovery, reducing caloric intake could help to reduce the risk of creating a caloric surplus that results in unnecessary weight gain. The additional rest, combined with planned recovery treatments such as an infrared sauna and foam rolling, are making a big difference in Allison's performance on race days. During a week when she is racing a 10K (6 mi), the additional calories help her maintain a steady pace throughout the entire race. During the week of a shorter race, she feels quicker and more energetic because she has consumed the exact amount of energy needed for her activities.

When you exercise at a moderate to high intensity for more than 50 or 60 minutes without consuming a sport drink or gel, you increase the risk that your body will use protein, rather than fat or carbohydrates, for fuel. When protein is used for fuel, not as much is available for tissue repair once the workout is complete. When you are going to be exercising at moderate to high intensity for more than 50 or 60 minutes, a sport drink could help ensure optimal carbohydrate use so that protein is conserved for tissue repair rather than used to fuel activity. Another risk of extended bouts of high-intensity exercise is that cortisol, produced to help ensure optimal fuel use during a workout, can also suppress the body's immune system; this means that an accumulation of stress, either from overtraining or other external sources, could actually weaken immunity.

The hormones epinephrine and norepinephrine work together to produce energy and regulate cardiorespiratory function during exercise. They are often referred to as adrenaline because they are produced by the adrenal gland. Once the body starts exercising, the physical stress signals the hypothalamus to release epinephrine and norepinephrine from the adrenal gland to elevate cardiac output, dilate blood vessels to enhance blood flow, increase blood glucose to help fuel exercise, and support the metabolism of FFAs into ATP. Glucagon, epinephrine, norepinephrine, and cortisol work together to increase circulating glucose before and during exercise (Kenney, Wilmore, and Costill 2022). The amount of glucose released by the liver and epinephrine produced by the adrenal gland depends on the intensity and duration of exercise.

Table 9.2 summarizes the production and functions of seven hormones related to metabolism.

TABLE 9.2 Primary Metabolic Hormones and Their Function

GLAND/ORGAN	HORMONE	STIMULUS	FUNCTIONS
Adrenal medulla (inner adrenal cortex)	Epinephrine	Physical stress (exercise) or emotional stress	Increases heart rate; increases blood sugar levels by breaking down glycogen (glycolysis); is involved in fat metabolism for energy
	Norepinephrine		Functions as a neurotransmitter to facilitate nerve signals and constrict blood vessels, which increases blood pressure
Adrenal cortex (outer adrenal cortex)	Cortisol (glucocorticoid)	Physical stress (exercise) or emotional stress	Releases FFAs to be metabolized into ATP for energy (fat metabolism); suppresses the immune system; conserves glucose by converting protein to ATP (gluconeogenesis); inhibits protein synthesis
Pancreas	Insulin	Elevated levels of blood glucose	Reduces blood glucose levels by promoting storage of glucose (as glycogen) in muscle cells and the liver
	Glucagon	Reduced levels of blood glucose	Elevates levels of blood glucose to provide energy for exercise
Stomach	Ghrelin	Released to stimulate hunger in response to glucose levels	Stimulates hunger signals; increases acid secretion for digestion
Adipose tissue (body fat)	Leptin	Insulin levels	Signals satiety (the feeling of being full)

Abbreviations: ATP, adenosine triphosphate; FFAs, free fatty acids.

Resistance and Sensitivity

Many hormones are released in bursts in response to specific stimuli; glands will release hormones in response to a chemical signal received by receptors or direct neural stimulation. For example, the body will not automatically elevate cortisol to make FFAs available for exercise; rather, a physical stress is the catalyst that stimulates cortisol to be released by the adrenal cortex. The release of cortisol then stimulates the subsequent release of FFAs to be metabolized into fuel. Hormone sensitivity means that an ample number of receptors are available in cells to allow a hormone to function efficiently. For example, strength training can improve the ability of type II muscle cells to convert glucose to ATP, resulting in improved insulin sensitivity, which is the ability of insulin to transport glucose to muscle cells. Conversely, a hormone is said to experience resistance when there are not enough receptors available in cells to react with it. As a result, the hormone won't be able to perform its function efficiently. For example, obesity could result in leptin resistance, which occurs when there are fewer receptor cells for leptin to interact with once it is produced to suppress hunger. In fact, research has shown that insulin resistance and abdominal obesity are associated with low-soluble leptin concentrations (Meier and Gressner 2004).

Chronic insulin resistance could result in type 2 diabetes, a disease in which the cells in muscles, fat, and the liver do not respond well to insulin. This causes the pancreas to make more insulin, but it is not able to produce enough to promote effective uptake of blood glucose into cells. Regular exercise, such as strength training, can enhance insulin sensitivity by promoting an increase of receptor cells that allow the hormone to function. Conversely, a sedentary lifestyle could result in insulin resistance, which means there are fewer receptor sites where the hormone can perform its intended function.

Macronutrients

The digestive system metabolizes macronutrients—protein, carbohydrates, and fat—to facilitate tissue repair, provide energy, and support optimal physiological function. A diet for optimal recovery should provide enough macronutrients to fuel all physical activity and support a healthy endocrine system.

The Role of Protein

Protein is the primary structural component of brain, nerve, blood, skin, and hair cells. The main function of the protein that you eat is to build and repair cells, including the muscle damage caused by exercising to the point of fatigue. Additional roles that dietary proteins play in the body include transporting cells, serving as enzymes to support various physiological functions, and acting as hormones.

While the primary role of protein is to repair damaged tissues, it can also be used to produce energy for muscle contractions when other sources of ATP (the cellular form of energy), namely fats and carbohydrates, are not available. *Gluconeogenesis* is the term that describes the conversion of protein to glycogen for ATP; however, this only occurs as the result of moderate- to high-intensity exercise that lasts for an extended period. Consuming sport drinks that contain sugar and sodium helps to maintain glycogen levels and avoid gluconeogenesis, sparing protein so it can be used to repair tissues after exercise. Limiting the duration of high-intensity activity to no more than 45 or 50 minutes can also help ensure an adequate supply of glycogen during exercise.

Amino acids are the building blocks of protein (*amino* means *containing nitrogen*). There are 20 amino acids; of these, 5 are considered nonessential because they can be produced by the body, 9 are essential because they cannot be produced in the body and must be consumed in the diet, and 6 are considered conditional—they can become essential, at which point they must be consumed in the diet. Consuming amino acids before and during a workout, combined with a postexercise recovery snack or meal containing protein, can increase muscle protein synthesis (the repair of muscle fibers damaged during exercise), which helps to promote overall recovery. Using a supplement with amino acids and proteins both before and during a high-intensity workout helps promote the recovery process once exercise is completed.

Protein provides about four calories of energy per gram. When consumed as part of a well-balanced diet, it can help provide a feeling of satiety, or being full, which can reduce feelings of hunger that could lead to consuming too many calories. In addition, protein is more energy expensive, meaning that compared with carbohydrates and fats, proteins require more energy during the digestive process, adding to the calories burned via the thermic effect of food.

As shown in table 9.3, the nutrition guidelines for protein consumption for an average, healthy adult are 0.8 to 1.0 grams of protein per kilogram of body weight (0.01 to 0.02 oz/lb). If you do a lot of aerobic endurance training, the recommended daily intake is 1.0 to 1.6 grams per kilogram of body weight (0.02 to 0.03 oz/lb). If you do a lot of strength training, then consuming 1.4 to 1.7 grams per kilogram of body weight (0.02 to 0.03 oz/lb) will support muscle protein synthesis—the repair of damaged proteins.

The body is constantly building new cells to replace old ones, and the protein you eat supports this process; 15 to 30 percent of your daily caloric intake should be protein, adjusted based on activity levels (specifically, the amount of strenuous activity or exercise), with more protein consumed on days of higher-intensity activity. For example, an active male with a body weight of 190 pounds (86 kg) who exercises at a moderate to vigorous intensity most days of the week should attempt to consume approximately 120 to 146 grams (4 to 5 oz) of protein per day, consumed throughout the day.

Protein quality varies. Casein, egg, milk, whey, and soy contain all of the essential amino acids and are easily digested and absorbed. Fruits, vegetables, grains, and nuts are incomplete proteins and must be combined during the day to ensure adequate intake of each of the essential amino acids. Casein and whey proteins are found in many common nutritional supplements. Whey protein is found in the liquid remaining after milk has been curdled and strained; it can be rapidly digested and could stimulate muscle protein synthesis more effectively than casein or soy. Casein is the protein that gives milk its white color and accounts for the majority of milk protein; it is slowly digested, which results in a prolonged release of amino acids.

TABLE 9.3 Protein Consumption Based on Body Weight

ACTIVITY	PROTEIN, G/KG BODY WEIGHT	PROTEIN, OZ/LB BODY WEIGHT
Average, healthy adult	0.8-1.0	0.01-0.02
Endurance athlete	1.0-1.6	0.02-0.03
Strength-oriented athlete	1.4-1.7	0.02-0.03

Adapted from Haff and Triplett (2016).

Applying the recommended guidelines to the previous example of a 190-pound (86 kg) active man, a good approach toward getting enough protein to promote muscle growth would be to consume 20 to 40 grams (0.7 to 1.4 oz) of protein at one time, distributed among three meals and two snacks.

The Role of Carbohydrates

Carbohydrates are stored as long chains of glucose molecules, called glycogen. Your body has the storage capacity of about 90 grams (3 oz) in the liver and 150 grams (5 oz) in muscle (Kenney, Wilmore, and Costill 2022). When energy is needed for muscle activity, glycogen stored in muscle and liver cells is first converted to glucose through a process called glycogenolysis before it is metabolized into ATP. During exercise, glycogen stored in muscle and liver cells or glucose circulating in the blood can be directed to working muscle cells.

When evaluating the quality of carbohydrates, the glycemic index and fiber content are two important considerations. Fiber serves many important and beneficial roles in the human body. High-viscosity fibers (formerly referred to as soluble fiber) include psyllium seeds, gums (found in foods like oats, legumes, guar, and barley), and pectin (found in foods like apples, citrus fruits, strawberries, and carrots). Slow gastric emptying, or the passage of food from the stomach into the intestines, helps to increase feelings of fullness; delayed gastric emptying slows the release of sugar into the bloodstream, which may help attenuate insulin resistance and can interfere with the absorption of fat and cholesterol and the recirculation of cholesterol in the liver, which may decrease cholesterol levels.

Low-viscosity fibers (previously referred to as insoluble fiber) include cellulose (found in whole-wheat flour, bran, and vegetables), hemicellulose (found in whole grains and bran), and lignin (found in mature vegetables, wheat, and fruit with edible seeds, such as strawberries and kiwi). Low-viscosity fibers play an important role in increasing fecal bulk and creating a laxative effect.

Carbohydrates provide about four calories of energy per gram for muscle contractions; they are metabolized into glucose (when transported through the blood) and glycogen (when stored in the liver and muscle cells). High-intensity exercise relies on glycogen to produce ATP. When muscles deplete stored glycogen, they can no longer perform as expected. One benefit of high-intensity exercise performed on a consistent basis is that muscle cells become more efficient at storing glycogen for future use. When stored in muscle tissue, 1 gram (0.04 oz) of glycogen holds 2.6 grams (0.09 fl oz) of water; as your muscles become more efficient at storing glycogen, they also store more water, which can lead to an increase in muscle size (Kenney, Wilmore, and Costill 2022). If you are training to compete in aerobic endurance events, this can allow you to store more energy for your competitions. However, if your goal is weight loss, then training your muscles to store glycogen (and water) could keep you from reaching a desired body weight. Table 9.4 lists the various amounts of carbohydrate needed for different training efforts.

It is possible to train muscles to store more glycogen prior to an endurance event. Yes, body weight can increase slightly in the short run, but the benefit is having more energy available to fuel a specific activity. One carbohydrate-loading protocol is to increase carbohydrate intake as training volume increases. Once the taper starts (approximately five to seven days before the event), continue eating the same amount of carbohydrates as before the taper, even though you are running fewer miles and at a slower pace. Because your running volume is decreasing, your muscle cells will store the additional glycogen (and water), leaving you with more fuel in your tank for your event (Kenney, Wilmore, and Costill 2022).

TABLE 9.4 Daily Carbohydrate Needs for Fueling and Recovery

DAILY NEEDS FOR FUELING AND RECOVERY		
SITUATION	**DESCRIPTION**	**CARBOHYDRATE TARGETS**
Light training load	Low-intensity or skill-based activities	3-5 g/kg (0.05-0.08 oz/lb) body weight per day
Moderate training load	Moderate exercise program (about 1 hr/day)	5-7 g/kg (0.08-0.11 oz/lb) body weight per day
High training load	Aerobic endurance program (1-3 hr/day of moderate- to high-intensity exercise)	6-10 g/kg (0.10-0.16 oz/lb) body weight per day
Very high training load	High-intensity speed, strength, and/or power training for competition (>4-5 hr/day of moderate- to high-intensity exercise)	8-12 g/kg (0.13-0.19 oz/lb) body weight per day
ACUTE FUELING STRATEGIES		
SITUATION	**DESCRIPTION**	**CARBOHYDRATE TARGETS**
General fueling up	Preparation for events involving <90 min exercise	7-12 g/kg (0.11-0.19 oz/lb) body weight for daily energy needs for 24 hr
Carbohydrate loading	Preparation for events involving >90 min sustained or intermittent exercise	10-12 g/kg (0.16-0.19 oz/lb) body weight per day for 36-48 hr
Pre-event fueling	Before exercise lasting >60 min	1-4 g/kg (0.02-0.06 oz/lb) body weight, consumed 1-4 hr before exercise Timing, amount, and type of carbohydrate foods and drinks are chosen to suit the practical needs of the event and individual preferences and experiences
During brief exercise	<45 min	Not needed
During sustained high-intensity exercise	45-75 min	Frequent 5- to 10-sec contact of the mouth and oral cavity with carbohydrate to promote central nervous system benefits
During aerobic endurance exercise, including start-and-stop sports	1-2.5 hr	30-60 g (1-2 oz) per hr to provide a source of muscle fuel to supplement endogenous stores
During ultra-endurance exercise	>2.5-3 hr	Up to 90 g (3 oz) per hr to support greater reliance on exogenous carbohydrate stores, using products providing multiple transportable carbohydrates (glucose–fructose mixtures) to achieve high rates of oxidation of carbohydrate consumed during exercise

Adapted by permission from L.M. Burke and E.S. Rawson, "Fueling and Nutrition," in *NSCA's Essentials of Sport Science,* edited for the National Strength and Conditioning Association by D.N. French and L.T. Ronda (Champaign, IL: Human Kinetics, 2022); Adapted from Thomas, Erdman, and Burke (2016).

The Role of Fat

Fat is not a four-letter word (literally or figuratively). However, many consider it a dirty word when it comes to nutrition, fitness, and exercise. For those who can remember the 1990s, you no doubt recall that a major marketing trend of the industrial food complex was to market and promote everything as low fat under the guise that it was a healthier option. (For those who don't remember that era, replace the current *gluten free*, *keto*, or *paleo* logos with *low fat* or *no fat* and you'll have the idea.) When it comes to our health, having high levels of body fat can be a risk factor for many types of chronic diseases; besides training for a favorite activity, an important reason to exercise is to reduce unhealthy, unnecessary fat to achieve and maintain a healthy body weight. However, as it relates to fueling and supporting optimal performance, fat, specifically the right kinds of fat, is an essential component of healthy nutrition.

The terms *fat*, *free fatty acids (FFAs)*, and *lipids* are used interchangeably when referring to fat metabolism. Lipids include triglycerides, which are formed by combining a glycerol with three fatty acids; most lipids in food and the body are in the form of triglycerides. Fat can be stored in skeletal muscle, the liver, and adipose tissue and is used for many functions, including providing structure for cell membranes, insulating and protecting vital organs, regulating endocrine system function (how hormones are produced), helping transport vitamins and minerals around the body, and acting as a source of energy for many cellular functions.

Fats (lipids) also serve as a ready source of stored energy, protect vital organs and bones, act as a means of absorption for fat-soluble vitamins, and produce hormones and cell membrane structures, among other necessary roles. Fat contains carbon, hydrogen, and oxygen atoms. Because fatty-acid chains have more carbon and hydrogen relative to oxygen, they yield more energy per gram: Fat provides nine calories of energy per gram, whereas protein and carbohydrates each deliver four calories per gram. Free fatty acids are the primary source of energy for the body while at rest and during low-intensity activity, which includes the postexercise recovery process.

One reason why your metabolism stays elevated after high-intensity exercise is that your muscles are still expending energy via aerobic metabolism, using FFAs. Lipolysis is the breakdown of triglycerides into a glycerol and three fatty acids for the purpose of producing ATP. When the body needs energy for physical activity, the hormones norepinephrine and cortisol act with receptor cells in adipose tissue to release the enzyme lipoprotein lipase, which breaks up triglycerides into the FFAs used by the mitochondria during a process called beta-oxidation. This ultimately results in the production of ATP. The result is that the three fatty acids and one glycerol of a single triglyceride can produce 457 molecules of ATP. For comparison, glycolysis (the conversion of glycogen to ATP) yields 36 to 39 ATP molecules per one unit of glucose (Kenney, Wilmore, and Costill 2022). Lipolysis is a slow process, which explains why it is the dominant source of energy during periods of rest or low-intensity physical activities. Glycolysis provides ATP more quickly, making it the go-to choice for ATP during moderate- to high-intensity physical activities.

Fatty Acids

There are four categories of fatty acids, which are long hydrocarbon chains with an even number of carbon atoms and varying degrees of saturation with hydrogen; these are classified as saturated, monounsaturated, polyunsaturated, and trans fats. Saturated fatty acids contain hydrogen on the carbon bonds, and because the body can produce these fats on its own, there are no dietary requirements for the consumption of saturated fats. Unsaturated fats contain double-carbon bonds with fewer hydrogen molecules; FFAs with one double-carbon bond are called monounsaturated, whereas fatty acids with two or more carbon bonds are polyunsaturated. The human body requires fatty acids of differing chain lengths and saturation to meet structural and metabolic needs.

Saturated Fats

Saturated fatty acids contain no double bonds between carbon atoms, are typically solid at room temperature, and are very stable, giving them a long shelf life. Saturated fat increases levels of low-density lipoprotein (LDL) cholesterol, considered the bad type of cholesterol because of its atherosclerotic properties. Saturated fats can be found in animal, dairy, and packaged food products and in coconut and palm kernel oils. Diets high in saturated fats are a risk factor for heart disease.

Unsaturated Fats

Unsaturated fatty acids contain one or more double bonds between carbon atoms, are typically liquid at room temperature, and are fairly unstable, making them susceptible to oxidative damage and reduced shelf life. The main form of monounsaturated fat is oleic acid; monounsaturated fats can be found in olive, peanut, and canola oils. Polyunsaturated fats include the essential (meaning they must be consumed in the diet) omega-3 fatty acids, found in many types of cold-water fish, and omega-6 fatty acids, found in soybean, corn, and safflower oils as well as foods made with those oils. Other foods that contain polyunsaturated and monounsaturated fats include avocados, flax and chia seeds, and almonds.

Polyunsaturated Fats

Polyunsaturated fats are important for optimal health. Substituting saturated fats or refined carbohydrates with polyunsaturated fats could reduce the risk of cardiovascular disease. Omega-3 fatty acids reduce blood clotting, dilate blood vessels, and reduce inflammation; however, as mentioned previously, the body cannot produce these essential fatty acids. Omega-3 (linolenic) fatty acids come in three forms: alpha-linolenic acid (ALA), eicosapentaenoic acid (EPA), and docosahexaenoic acid (DHA), the type of omega-3 found in plants. Alpha-linolenic acid is converted to EPA and DHA in the body. Docosahexaenoic acid and EPA omega-3 fatty acids are naturally found in egg yolks as well as in cold-water fish and shellfish like tuna, salmon, mackerel, cod, crab, shrimp, and oysters. They are important for eye and brain development (and are especially important for a growing fetus in the late stages of pregnancy); they also act to reduce cholesterol and triglyceride levels and may help to preserve brain function and reduce the risk of mental illness and attention-deficit hyperactivity disorder. Omega-6 fatty acid (linoleic acid) is generally consumed in abundance; it is an essential fatty acid found in flaxseed, canola, and soybean oils and in green, leafy vegetables.

Trans Fats

Trans fats are made when an unsaturated fat, normally liquid at room temperature, is hydrogenated (hydrogen atoms are added) so that it turns into a solid. This manufacturing process increases the shelf life of a food product, explaining why many packaged foods can be high in trans fats. However, because it changes the chemical structure of fat, trans fat has been linked to heart disease and elevated levels of LDL cholesterol.

The process of making a trans fat involves breaking the double bond of the unsaturated fat and forming an altered unsaturated fat, referred to as a synthetic or industrial trans fat (a transformation from the "cis" formation to a "trans" formation, thus the name *trans fat*). Hydrogenation is the process of converting an unsaturated fatty acid to a saturated fatty acid by replacing the double bonds with hydrogen. Both partial hydrogenation and full hydrogenation cause changes to cell membrane fluidity and negatively affect cell function. Synthetic trans fats significantly elevate LDL cholesterol and are implicated in the development and progression of cardiovascular disease. Many cooking oils still contain notable amounts of trans fat; check the ingredients for partially hydrogenated oils to determine if a food contains trans fat in order to reduce your intake.

Fat Is Energy

Ultimately, fat is an important source of energy, fat-soluble vitamins, and essential fatty acids. The myth of the fat-burning zone (exercise at about 60 to 70 percent of the maximum heart rate) is not really a myth; lipolysis, the breaking down of fats to release energy, requires oxygen, which is readily available during lower-intensity physical activities. Muscles primarily use fat as the source of ATP during low-intensity activity. (However, as the intensity of exercise increases, the demand for energy is greater, and the working muscles will need ATP more quickly than lipolysis can provide, so higher-intensity exercise ultimately burns more calories.) Eating adequate amounts and types of healthy fats can definitely play an important role in supporting postexercise recovery.

Timing Your Fuel

High-intensity exercise depletes energy and damages tissues. Therefore, on the days you know you will be pushing your body to the limit, it is important to adjust your nutrition to address your specific needs. Nutrition can be extremely personal, and there are a number of eating strategies you could follow to consume your daily requirements; the important thing is that when you consistently exercise at a high intensity, proper nutrition is a component of the recovery process. Proper nutrition is essential for getting the most out of your workout and recovery programs; further, it's not just what you eat but also when you eat that can help promote recovery from high-intensity exercise. When it comes to your nutrition, eating the proper amount of food at the right time can ensure optimal fuel for your workouts; nutrient timing is the concept that *when* macronutrients are consumed relative to exercise is as important, if not more so, than *what* is actually consumed. The right types and amounts of food before, during, and after exercise can maximize the amount of energy available to fuel optimal performance, minimize the amount of gastrointestinal distress, and support postexercise glycogen replenishment and protein synthesis. As Arent and colleagues (2020) observed in their review of the topic,

The period following exercise provides an ideal opportunity for timed nutrient intake in order to promote the restoration of muscle glycogen and protein synthesis, while helping to reduce muscle protein breakdown. . . . Post-exercise nutrient timing may be an essential aspect of an optimal training program as it has the potential to improve the rate of recovery and maximizes training adaptations (8).

Nutrient Timing: Position Statement From the International Society of Sports Nutrition

The International Society of Sports Nutrition (ISSN) provides an objective and critical review regarding the timing of macronutrients in relation to healthy exercise for adults, and in particular, information for highly trained individuals on exercise performance and body composition. The following points summarize the position of the ISSN (Kersick et al. 2017):

- Nutrient timing incorporates the use of methodical planning and eating of whole foods, fortified foods, and dietary supplements. The timing of energy intake and the ratio of certain ingested macronutrients may enhance recovery and tissue repair, augment muscle protein synthesis, and improve mood state after a high volume of intense exercise.

- Endogenous glycogen stores are maximized by following a high-carbohydrate diet (8 to 12 grams of carbohydrate per kilogram of body mass [0.1 to 0.2 oz/lb]); moreover, these stores are depleted most by high-volume exercise.

- If rapid restoration of glycogen is required (recovery time is less than four hours), then the following strategies should be considered:
  - Aggressive carbohydrate replenishing (1.2 grams per kilogram of body weight [0.02 oz/lb] per hour), with a preference toward carbohydrate sources that have a high glycemic index (greater than 70)
  - The addition of caffeine (3 to 8 milligrams per kilogram of body weight [1 to 4 mg/lb])
  - Combining carbohydrates (0.8 grams per kilogram of body weight [0.01 oz/lb] per hour) with protein (0.2 to 0.4 grams per kilogram of body weight [0.003 to 0.006 oz/lb] per hour)

- Extended (longer than 60 minutes) bouts of high-intensity exercise (more than 70 percent of the $\dot{V}O_2max$) challenge fuel supply and fluid regulation; thus, carbohydrates should be consumed at a rate of approximately 30 to 60 grams (1 to 2 oz) of carbohydrate per hour in a 6- to 8-percent carbohydrate–electrolyte solution (6 to 12 fluid ounces [177 to 355 mL]) every 10 to 15 minutes throughout the entire exercise bout, particularly during exercise bouts that extend beyond 70 minutes. When carbohydrate delivery is inadequate, adding protein may help increase performance, ameliorate muscle damage, promote euglycemia, and facilitate glycogen resynthesis.

Strategies to fuel vigorous exercise should address three specific stages: pre-exercise, exercise, and postexercise. The two main functions of a pre-exercise snack are to optimize glucose availability and glycogen stores and to provide the fuel needed for exercise performance. The goal of fueling while you are exercising is to maintain optimal blood glucose levels so that muscle cells have access to immediate energy. It can take about four to six hours to properly digest a meal; therefore, on the day of an athletic competition or intense workout, it is import-

- Carbohydrate ingestion throughout resistance exercise (i.e., three to six sets of the 8- to 12-repetition maximum using multiple exercises targeting all major muscle groups) has been shown to promote euglycemia and higher glycogen stores. Consuming carbohydrates solely or in combination with protein during resistance training increases muscle glycogen stores, ameliorates muscle damage, and facilitates greater acute and chronic training adaptations.
- Meeting the total daily intake of protein, preferably with evenly spaced protein consumption (approximately every three hours during the day), should be viewed as a primary area of emphasis for exercising individuals.
- Ingestion of essential amino acids (approximately 10 grams [0.4 oz]), either in free form or as part of a protein bolus of approximately 20 to 40 grams (0.7 to 1.4 oz), has been shown to maximally stimulate muscle protein synthesis.
- Pre-exercise and postexercise nutritional interventions (carbohydrate plus protein or protein alone) may operate as an effective strategy to support increases in strength and improvements in body composition. However, the size and timing of a pre-exercise meal may affect the extent to which postexercise nutrition is required.
- Ingestion of high-quality protein sources immediately to two hours after exercise stimulates robust increases in muscle protein synthesis.
- In nonexercising scenarios, changing the frequency of meals has been shown to have a limited effect on weight loss and body composition, with stronger evidence to indicate that meal frequency can favorably improve appetite and satiety. More research is needed to determine how combining an exercise program with altered meal frequencies influences weight loss and body composition, but preliminary research indicates a potential benefit.
- Ingesting a 20- to 40-gram (0.7 to 1.4 oz) dose (0.25 to 0.40 grams per kilogram of body mass [0.004 to 0.006 oz/lb] per dose) of a high-quality protein source every three to four hours appears to most favorably affect muscle protein synthesis rates when compared with other dietary patterns and is associated with improved body composition and performance outcomes.
- Consuming casein protein (approximately 30 to 40 grams [1.1 to 1.4 oz]) prior to sleep can increase muscle protein synthesis and metabolic rate throughout the night without influencing lipolysis.

Adapted from Kersick, Arent, Schoenfeld, et al. (2017).

ant to prepare and plan your meals so you allow time for digestion before being physically active. Once a preworkout meal has been digested and absorbed, liver and muscle glycogen levels are at their highest. As you train, it is a good idea to experiment with preworkout meals and their timing so you can identify the optimal food and when to eat for a full tank of gas.

Keep in mind that when you exercise for longer than 50 or 60 minutes, blood glucose levels will start to drop, and you might feel like your batteries are being drained. Therefore, as a general rule when training for an endurance event that lasts longer than an hour, you should try different combinations of snacks and drinks to identify the optimal source of fuel while you are exercising. That way, you can practice fueling while you train so you know how to optimize performance through nutrition on competition day.

Sleep, the Ultimate Recovery Method

Sleep is one of the most effective methods for recovering from a hard workout and is one healthy lifestyle habit that you are already doing, but you may not be getting the correct amount or quality of sleep, and therefore, you may not wake up fully rested. As mentioned in chapter 6, a surefire method of promoting recovery so that your workouts produce the desired results is to achieve optimal sleep. "I'll get enough sleep when I'm dead" is a common sentiment stated by people who fill their schedules with both work and social commitments, but the reality is that not getting enough sleep *could* result in an early death, making it a self-fulfilling prophecy. Evidence suggests that insufficient sleep is a risk factor for obesity, diabetes, cardiovascular diseases, depression, impaired driving, and more (Chennaoui et al. 2014).

After completing a high-intensity workout, sleep is when your body will continue its return to complete homeostasis. Achieving results from exercise requires getting the optimal quality and quantity of sleep. You work hard in the gym and pay close attention to your nutrition, yet if you're not focusing the same level of effort on your sleep, you may not be getting the results you want. Improving both the quality and quantity of your sleep not only could help you recover more effectively, it could improve your overall health. Sleep allows muscles to repair damaged tissues and replace spent energy. The best thing about using sleep to enhance recovery from exercise is that there are no additional costs!

Circadian Rhythms and Weight

Circadian rhythms determine the body's innate sense of time and how hormones respond to levels of light and darkness. As the sun goes down, the circadian rhythms will naturally start preparing the body for sleep; exposure to light sources such as electronic screens, a stressful situation, hunger, or substances such as caffeine, sugar, or alcohol could interrupt the body's ability to transition to sleep. Melatonin is a hormone that lowers the body's temperature in preparation for sleep; too much light in the evening or during nighttime could lower melatonin production, thus making it harder to fall asleep. When you're unsuccessfully trying to fall asleep, your body might think it needs energy and starts releasing cortisol to stimulate energy production, making it difficult to fall asleep even when you feel tired. If you struggle to fall asleep, limiting screen time in the later evening hours to allow circadian rhythms to be more aligned with the natural light cycle could help. If you find that you have a hard time falling asleep, even when you feel physically tired, then it might be necessary to examine your evening routine to identify simple adjustments that could result in better sleep hygiene. In addition to reducing overall stress and helping to lower cortisol levels, increasing the quantity and quality of sleep could also help you to regulate metabolic hormones, which is essential for achieving and maintaining a healthy body weight.

For both men and women, sleeping less than six hours per night could result in higher levels of belly fat. A lack of sleep can elevate activity of the sympathetic nervous system, which is responsible for stimulating the metabolism to produce the energy for physical activity. Insufficient sleep could elevate levels of the hormones cortisol and epinephrine, which help release FFAs to be used for energy; when there is insufficient physical activity, the FFAs can be deposited in the adipose tissue of the abdominal region, resulting in additional belly fat (Kenney, Wilmore, and Costill 2022).

Another way that insufficient sleep could lead to weight gain is through the production of ghrelin and leptin, hormones that stimulate hunger and tell the body when it has had enough food intake, respectively. Poor sleep has been associated with an imbalance in these hormones, which could result in overeating (Chennaoui et al. 2014). Plus, staying awake late into the evening allows more opportunities for mindless snacking on calorie-dense food.

Stages of Sleep

If you are looking for an immediate performance enhancer, consider getting more and better sleep. Making the effort to improve both the quality and quantity of your sleep can have an almost immediate effect on your performance. While you are sleeping, your body can experience multiple cycles of sleep, each of which can last between 70 and 120 minutes; there are three stages of non-rapid-eye-movement (non-REM) sleep and a fourth stage of rapid-eye-movement (REM) sleep (Bushman 2013). Practicing proper sleep hygiene means creating an environment where you are able to cycle through the following four stages of non-REM and REM sleep so you can wake up properly refreshed with an adequate supply of energy.

1. *Stage 1: Non-REM.* The body has just dozed off and is preparing to enter stage 2; this stage can last between one and five minutes.

2. *Stage 2: Non-REM.* The body is essentially powering down by reducing activity in the brain and body; this stage can last between 10 and 60 minutes.

3. *Stage 3: Non-REM.* Brain activity slows down and relaxes; this stage can last between 20 and 40 minutes.

4. *Stage 4: REM.* Activity in the brain increases while most of the body experiences temporary paralysis so that your muscles don't react to any visual stimulation you may experience while dreaming; REM sleep can last between 10 and 60 minutes.

Maintaining Good Sleep Hygiene

Despite the amount of research on the subject, scientists and medical professionals who study sleep are not sure why we need it. However, it is well established that achieving optimal sleep is essential for long-term health. The Sleep Foundation provides the following suggestions for how to improve sleep habits (Suni 2022):

- Keep a regular sleep schedule. Try to go to bed at the same time every night.
- Sleep in a dark room. Remove the television and leave electronic screens in another room. The bedroom should be for sleeping, not watching television.
- Don't eat right before bed; digestion could interrupt the process of falling asleep.
- Reduce overall levels of stress. This is easier said than done, but regular exercise plays an important role in reducing stress levels.

Making a specific effort to develop habits like getting optimal sleep can make a big difference in being able to achieve and maintain a state of physical preparedness. The great news is that as you improve your sleep habits, you should start seeing better results from your workouts, especially if you are properly recording and tracking your efforts.

Meditation

The word *meditation* may conjure images of either a room full of yoga enthusiasts sitting quietly in awkward positions or a group of spiritual practitioners chanting in rhythm, not an executive in a power suit or a soldier outfitted with weapons of war. However, professional athletes do it. Business executives do it. Even military special operators do it. In recent years, high performers in a number of different fields have all begun participating in the practice of meditation. Yes, meditation may play an important role in a religious practice or be an integral component of a yoga class, but it can also help promote recovery after exercise. Think of the brain as a muscle and meditation as a form of exercise to make it stronger. You know that lifting weights can make your muscles stronger, or that logging those miles can improve your aerobic capacity, so why not learn more about meditation so you can use it to speed up the return to homeostasis?

Understanding Meditation

For centuries, meditation has played an important role in many religious rituals. It's still a component of many spiritual practices, and now, due to the ability to measure brain waves, modern science can quantify specific physiological benefits of meditation, which has helped promote the practice outside of the traditional settings. First, it is important to understand what meditation is as well as what it is not. Meditation is the ability to quiet the mind in order to let go of distracting thoughts and focus attention on the present moment. In an exercise environment, meditation is often performed as a final component of a yoga class; however, it can be practiced during any type of workout, if you are intentional about making the time for it. Although yoga and meditation have been traditionally classified as modes of mind–body exercise, it's important to understand that *any* time you are moving, it is technically a mind–body exercise, because you have to focus on what you are doing in the moment. When we move, we are often doing so for a purpose and need to concentrate on what we are doing so we can move with precision and coordination. Unlike other modes of exercise, where an established form or technique is important and can make a difference in the outcome, there is not one specific way to meditate. Successful meditation merely requires the ability to slow down, breathe deeply, relax the mind, and bring awareness to the present moment.

This means that meditation doesn't need to happen from a specific posture or body position, and it can certainly happen as the body is moving. Exercise itself can be a form of meditation through movement, because you have to focus exactly on what you are doing in that precise moment so you can complete the exercise with the lowest risk of injury possible. For example, exercise like running or hiking could be considered dynamic meditation, because to achieve success, it is necessary to develop a strong mind–body connection that is capable of removing distracting thoughts while being fully engaged in the present moment and participating in the activity.

The fundamental purpose of meditation is to bring awareness to what you are doing and how you are feeling in a specific moment, and there are different meditation methods that can be practiced during or after a high-intensity workout. Juan Carlos Santana, owner of the Institute of Human Performance in Boca Raton, Florida, and a strength coach who works with clients ranging from professional mixed martial artists to older adults who want to remain active through their golden years, believes that meditation is essential in a fitness program and practices a unique approach that he calls "present moment awareness" with his clients (McCall 2018). As he explains,

> I encourage my athletes to be present in the moment so they can improve their performance by concentrating on whatever task is challenging them at *that* moment. In my experience, people will quit a physical challenge based on what they fear *WILL* happen, which is projecting into the future, as opposed to what is actually happening in the present, the now. During our workouts, I encourage my clients to relax their face—learning how to remove the grimace when doing hard exercise is the first step toward learning how to be present in the moment. If we can help our clients learn how to be comfortable when things get hard, we will be giving them skills that can be used in all aspects of their life, not just during a workout.

Likewise, group fitness instructors encourage class participants to incorporate meditation in their exercise programs. Clifton Harski, a personal trainer based in St. Louis, Missouri, describes how he likes to use meditation in the group workout programs he coaches:

> Meditation asks that you empty your mind and focus on breathing. At the beginning of the class, I encourage my class participants to empty their minds so they can focus on the physical tasks at hand. I want them to focus on the process of learning movement, which in itself can be a form of meditation (pers. comm.).

A meta-analysis of the existing research on meditation suggested that the practice does indeed produce quantifiable benefits. The comprehensive review of the literature identified two main findings: (1) Meditation has a substantial effect on psychological variables, and (2) its effects might be somewhat stronger for negative emotional variables as opposed to cognitive variables (Sedlmeier et al. 2012). Recognized benefits of meditation include the following:

- Enhanced concentration
- Reduced stress
- Less anxiety
- Feelings of calm
- Greater mental clarity

In recent years, science has been able to measure exactly how meditation influences the brain. One significant benefit that has been identified is the effect on the medial prefrontal cortex, the part of the brain that processes information relating specifically to the self (often referred to as the "me center"). When stress accumulates, it can influence this part of the brain, leading to the perception that things are happening directly to you on purpose, which can subsequently increase feelings of anxiety. Meditation can reduce activity in the medial prefrontal cortex while increasing activity in the lateral prefrontal cortex, the part of the brain that considers incoming information from a more logical perspective and is often referred to as the "assessment center." Regular meditation can reduce activity in the me center while engaging the assessment center, helping to control anxiety and allowing events to be perceived from a more rational, objective point of view (Gladding 2013).

Adding Meditation to Your Toolbox

In this day and age, when people are almost always multitasking and constantly checking social media for status updates or likes on their latest posts (we're all guilty of that), it seems like the ability to just simply sit and be quiet is a lost skill. Think about what happens when you find yourself waiting in a line for more than a few moments, whether at the local coffee shop or waiting for the exercise class ahead of yours to be over. You probably whip out your phone and start tapping the screen. However, consider small moments like this as perfect opportunities for brief meditation. In addition, meditation could be done while sitting in a sauna or performing static stretching by applying these simple steps:

1. Set a timer for 30 to 60 seconds.
2. Perform the stretch.
3. Relax your mind.
4. Breathe deeply.

Intentionally focus on the process of breathing while performing the stretch; once the timer goes off, move to the next muscle and repeat. This is a simple and effective way to combine the benefits of meditation and stretching at the same time.

The heart of meditation is the ability to take a break from the chaos of daily life to be still and focus on the self.

The following are some additional tips for how to practice meditation (Valley Health System 2017). Try these yourself, and as you find what works, add it to your normal workout program:

- Pay close attention to breathing.
- Notice what you're sensing in a given moment—the sights, sounds, and smells that ordinarily slip by without reaching your conscious awareness.
- Tune in to physical sensations. From your posture to the way the air is circulating around your body, focus inward to really notice what your body is feeling in this moment.

Returning to Homeostasis

Stress, regardless of the source, disrupts homeostasis. Exercise is a physical stress that involves all the major physiological systems of the body; the level of intensity and duration of the exercise will determine the disruption to homeostasis. Once exercise is over, the four general strategies that can help your body return to homeostasis are rest, rehydration, refueling, and tissue repair. Applying specific techniques from one of these general strategies could help you to accelerate the return to homeostasis once your workout is over. No matter what your fitness goals, you are probably spending more time in postworkout recovery than you are performing the actual exercises that change your body. As you design and plan the exercises for your workouts, look at the intensity and volume of your overall training program. Does it allow for enough rest between high-intensity workouts? Does it make postworkout tissue treatment a priority? Does it adjust the intensity of your workouts so you are performing relatively low-intensity workouts on the days after your hardest ones?

Getting results from exercise is not an exact science. Yes, we can perform experiments, monitor results, and identify trends, but each individual person is different, and we will each respond to exercise in our own way. Knowing how the stress of exercise disrupts your body down to the cellular level, combined with understanding how the benefits of rest, nutrition, and low-intensity exercise can promote the desired adaptations, makes you formidable, because not only do you know how exercise changes your body but you also know the power of rest and how to apply specific recovery strategies to allow the changes to occur. As you prepare your workouts, keep in mind that it may not be performing an extra set or repetition that could make the difference, but having the courage to *not* perform the extra work and instead allow more time for a complete rest. Remember, tomorrow's workout starts at the end of today's. How you refuel, rehydrate, rest, and allow your body to repair will determine how effectively you train. Choose wisely.

REFERENCES

Chapter 1

Bandyopadhyay, A., I. Bhattacharjee, and P.K. Sousana. 2012. "Physiological Perspective of Endurance Overtraining—A Comprehensive Update." *Al Ameen Journal of Medical Sciences* 5 (1): 7-20.

Bishop, P., E. Jones, and K. Woods. 2008. "Recovery From Training: A Brief Review." *Journal of Strength and Conditioning Research* 22 (3): 1015-24.

Cheng, A.J., B. Jude, and J.T. Lanner. 2020. "Intramuscular Mechanisms of Overtraining." *Redox Biology* 35: 221-30.

Department of Health and Human Services. 2018. *Physical Activity Guidelines for Americans*. 2nd ed. Washington, DC: Department of Health and Human Services.

Fry, A.C., W.J. Kraemer, F. van Borselen, J.M. Lynch, J.L. Marsit, E.P. Roy, N.T. Triplett, and H.T. Knuttgen. 1994. "Performance Decrements with High-Intensity Resistance Exercise Overtraining." *Medicine and Science in Sports and Exercise* 26: 1165-73.

Haff, G.G., and N.T. Triplett. 2016. *Essentials of Strength Training and Conditioning*. 4th ed. Champaign, IL: Human Kinetics.

Hausswirth, C., and I. Mujika, eds. 2013. *Recovery for Performance in Sport*. Champaign, IL: Human Kinetics.

Kenney, W.L., J.H. Wilmore, and D.L. Costill. 2022. *Physiology of Sport and Exercise*. 8th ed. Champaign, IL: Human Kinetics.

Meeusen, R., M. Duclos, C. Foster, A. Fry, M. Gleeson, D. Nieman, J. Raglin, G. Rietiens, J. Steinacker, and A. Urhausen. 2013. "Prevention, Diagnosis, and Treatment of the Over Training Syndrome: Joint Consensus Statement of the European College of Sports Medicine and the American College of Sports Medicine." *Medicine and Science in Sports and Exercise* 45: 186-205.

Sabia, S., A. Fayosse, J. Dumurgier, V. van Hees, C. Paquet, A. Sommerlad, M. Kivimaki, A. Dugravot, and A. Singh-Manoux. 2021. "Association of Sleep Duration in Middle and Old Age with Incidence of Dementia." *Nature Communications* 12: 2289. Accessed on December 31, 2021. https://www.nature.com/articles/s41467-021-22354-2.

Snyder, A.C., and A.C. Hackney. 2013. "The Endocrine System in Overtraining." In *Endocrinology of Physical Activity and Sport*, 2nd ed., edited by A.C. Hackney and N.W. Constantini, 524. New York: Springer.

Chapter 2

Bessa, A.L., V.N. Oliveira, G.G. Agostini, R.J.S. Oliveira, A.C.S. Oliveira, G.E. White, G.D. Wells, D.N.S. Teixeira, and F.S. Espindola. 2016. "Exercise Intensity and Recovery: Biomarkers of Injury, Inflammation and Oxidative Stress." *Journal of Strength and Conditioning Research* 30 (2): 311-19.

Bryant, C.X., S. Merrill, and D.J. Green, eds. 2014. *American Council on Exercise Personal Trainer Manual*. 5th ed. San Diego, CA: American Council on Exercise.

Cheng, A.J., B. Jude, and J.T. Lanner. 2020. "Intramuscular Mechanisms of Overtraining." *Redox Biology* 35: 221-30.

Eston, R. 2012. "Use of Ratings of Perceived Exertion in Sports." *International Journal of Sports Physiology and Performance* 12 (7): 175-82.

Haff, G.G., and N.T. Triplett. 2016. *Essentials of Strength Training and Conditioning.* 4th ed. Champaign, IL: Human Kinetics.

Kenney, W.L., J.H. Wilmore, and D.L. Costill. 2022. *Physiology of Sport and Exercise.* 8th ed. Champaign, IL: Human Kinetics.

McKee, J. 2013. "Tackling Rhabdomyolysis in College Football Players." *AAOS Now,* September 1, 2013. www.aaos.org/aaosnow/2013/sep/clinical/clinical4.

Robergs, R.A., and R. Landwehr. 2002. "The Surprising History of the 'HRmax=220-age' Equation." *Journal of Exercise Physiology* 5 (2). www.asep.org/asep/asep/Robergs2.pdf.

Sutton, B.G., ed. 2021. *NASM Essentials of Personal Fitness Training.* 7th ed. Burlington, MA: Jones and Bartlett Learning.

Chapter 3

Bishop, P.A., E. Jones, and A.K. Woods. 2008. "Recovery From Training: A Brief Review." *Journal of Strength and Conditioning Research* 22 (3): 1015-24.

Cheng, A.J., B. Jude, and J.T. Lanner. 2020. "Intramuscular Mechanisms of Overtraining." *Redox Biology* 35: 221-20.

Dupuy, O., W. Douzi, D. Theurot, L. Bosquet, and B. Dugue. 2018. "An Evidence-Based Approach for Choosing Post-Exercise Recovery Techniques to Reduce Markers of Muscle Damage, Soreness, Fatigue, and Inflammation: A Systemic Review with Meta-Analysis." *Frontiers in Physiology* 9 (403): 1-15.

Gleeson, M. 2007. "Immune Function in Sport and Exercise." *Journal of Applied Physiology* 103 (2): 693-99.

Haff, G.G., and N.T. Triplett. 2016. *Essentials of Strength Training and Conditioning.* 4th ed. Champaign, IL: Human Kinetics.

Halabchi, F., Z. Ahmadinejad, and M. Selk-Ghaffari. 2020. "COVID-19 Epidemic: Exercise or Not to Exercise; That Is the Question!" *Asian Journal of Sports Medicine,* March 2020.

Hausswirth, C., and I. Mujika. 2013. *Recovery for Performance in Sport.* Champaign, IL: Human Kinetics.

Hoffman, J. 2014. *Physiological Aspects of Sport Training and Performance.* 2nd ed. Champaign, IL: Human Kinetics.

Kenney, W.L., J.H. Wilmore, and D.L. Costill. 2022. *Physiology of Sport and Exercise.* 8th ed. Champaign, IL: Human Kinetics.

Lee, E.C., M.S. Fragala, S.A. Kavouras, R.M. Queen, J.L. Pryor, and D.J. Casa. 2017. "Biomarkers in Sports and Exercise: Tracking Health, Performance, and Recovery in Athletes." *The Journal of Strength and Conditioning Research* 31 (10): 2920-37.

Peake, J.M., O. Neubauer, N.P. Walsh, and R.J. Simpson. 2017. "Recovery of the Immune System After Exercise." *Journal of Applied Physiology* 122 (5): 1077-87.

Simpson, R.J., J.P. Campbell, M. Gleeson, K. Krüger, D.C. Nieman, D.B. Pyne, J.E. Turner, and N.P. Walsh. 2020. "Can Exercise Affect Immune Function to Increase Susceptibility to Infection?" *Exercise Immunology Review* 26: 8-22.

Simpson, R.J., H. Kunz, N. Agha, and R. Graff. 2015. "Exercise and the Regulation of Immune Functions." *Progress in Molecular Biology and Translational Science* 135: 355-80.

Snyder, A.C., and A.C. Hackney. 2013. "The Endocrine System in Overtraining." In *Endocrinology of Physical Activity and Sport*, 2nd ed., edited by A.C. Hackney and N.W. Constantini, 524. New York: Springer.

Wyatt, F.B., A. Donaldson, and E. Brown. 2013. "The Overtraining Syndrome: A Meta-analytic Review." *Journal of Exercise Physiology* 16 (2): 12-23.

Chapter 4

Bishop, P., E. Jones, and K. Woods. 2008. "Recovery From Training: A Brief Review." *Journal of Strength and Conditioning Research* 22 (3): 1015-24.

Chapter 5

Cook, G. 2010. *Movement: Functional Movement Systems*. Santa Cruz, CA: On Target.

Earls, J. 2014. *Born to Walk: Myofascial Efficiency and the Body in Movement*. Chichester, England: Lotus Publishing.

Galli, C., S. Guizzardi, G. Passeri, G.M. Macaluso, and R. Scandroglio. 2005. "Life on the Wire: On Tensegrity and Force Balance in Cells." *Acta BioMed* 76 (1): 512.

Healey, K., D. Hatfield, P. Blanpied, L. Dorfman, and D. Riebe. 2013. "The Effects of Myofascial Release With Foam Rolling on Performance." *Journal of Strength and Conditioning Research* 28 (1): 61-68.

Ingber, D.E. 2003. "Tensegrity II: How Structural Networks Influence Cellular Information Processing Networks." *Journal of Cell Science* 116: 1397-1408.

Ingber, D.E. 2004. "The Mechanochemical Basis of Cell and Tissue Regulation." *Mechanics and Chemistry of Biosystems* 1 (1): 53-68.

MacDonald, G.Z., D.C. Button, E.J. Drinkwater, and D.G. Behm. 2014. "Foam Rolling as a Recovery Tool After an Intense Bout of Physical Activity." *Medicine and Science in Sports and Exercise* 46 (1): 131-42.

MacDonald, G.Z., M.D.H. Penney, M.E. Mullaley, A.L. Cuconato, C.D.J. Drake, D.G. Behm, and D.C. Button. 2013. "An Acute Bout of Self-Myofascial Release Increases Range of Motion Without a Subsequent Decrease in Muscle Activation or Force." *Journal of Strength and Conditioning Research* 27 (3): 812-21.

Mauntel, T., M. Clark, and D. Padua. 2014. "Effectiveness of Myofascial Release Therapies on Physical Performance Measurements: A Systematic Review." *Athletic Training and Sports Health Care* 6 (4): 189-96.

Mohr, A.R., B.C. Long, and C.L. Goad. 2014. "Effect of Foam Rolling and Static Stretching on Passive Hip-Flexion Range of Motion." *Journal of Sport Rehabilitation* 23 (4): 296-99.

Myers, T. 2020. *Anatomy Trains: Myofascial Meridians for Manual and Movement Therapists*. 4th ed. London: Elsevier.

Neumann, D. 2010. *Kinesiology of the Musculoskeletal System*. 2nd ed. St. Louis, MO: Mosby.

Schleip, R. 2015. *Fascia in Sport and Movement*. Edinburgh, Scotland: Handspring Publishing.

Schleip, R. 2017. *Fascial Fitness: How to be Resilient, Elegant, and Dynamic in Everyday Life and Sport*. Chichester, England: Lotus Publishing.

Schleip, R., T.W. Findley, L. Chaitow, and P.A. Huijing, eds. 2012. *Fascia: The Tensional Network of the Human Body*. London: Elsevier.

Schultz, R.L., and R. Feitis. 1996. *The Endless Web: Fascial Anatomy and Physical Reality*. Berkeley, CA: North Atlantic Books.

Shah, S., and A. Bhalara. 2012. "Myofascial Release." *International Journal of Health Sciences and Research* 2 (2): 69-77.

Verkoshansky, Y., and M. Siff. 2009. *Supertraining*. 6th ed. Denver, CO: Supertraining Institute.

Vogel, V., and M. Sheetz. 2006. "Local Force and Geometry Sensing Regulate Cell Functions." *Nature Reviews: Molecular Cell Biology* (7): 265-75.

Chapter 6

Arent, S., H. Cintineo, B. McFadden, A. Chandler, and M. Arent. 2020. "Nutrient Timing: A Garage Door of Opportunity?" *Nutrients* 12 (7): 1948-67.

Born, D.P, B. Sperlich, and H.C. Holmberg. 2013. "Bringing Light into Dark: Effects of Compression Clothing on Performance and Recovery." *International Journal of Sports Physiology and Performance* 8 (1): 4-18.

Chennaoui, M., P. Arnal, F. Sauvet, and D. Leger. 2014. "Sleep and Exercise: A Reciprocal Issue?" *Sleep Medicine Reviews* 20: 59-72.

Duffield, R., J. Edge, R. Merrells, E. Hawke, M. Barnes, D. Simcock, and N. Gill. 2008. "The Effects of Compression Garments on Intermittent Exercise Performance and Recovery on Consecutive Days." *International Journal of Sports Physiology and Performance* 3 (4): 454-68.

Dupuy, O., W. Douzi, D. Theurot, L. Bosquet, and B. Dugue. 2018. "An Evidence-Based Approach for Choosing Post-Exercise Recovery Techniques to Reduce Markers of Muscle Damage, Soreness, Fatigue, and Inflammation: A Systemic Review with Meta-Analysis." *Frontiers in Physiology* 9 (403): 1-15.

Haff, G.G., and N.T. Triplett. 2016. *Essentials of Strength Training and Conditioning*. 4th ed. Champaign, IL: Human Kinetics.

Hausswirth, C., and I. Mujika. 2013. *Recovery for Performance in Sport*. Champaign, IL: Human Kinetics.

Kersick, C., S. Arent, B. Schoenfeld, J. Stout, B. Campbell, C. Wilborn, L. Taylor, et al. 2017. "International Society of Sports Nutrition Position Stand: Nutrient Timing." *Journal of the International Society of Sports Nutrition* 14: 33. https://doi.org/10.1186/s12970-017-0189-4.

LaForgia, J., R. Withers, and C. Gore. 2006. "Effects of Exercise Intensity and Duration on the Excess Post-Exercise Oxygen Consumption." *Journal of Sport Sciences* 24 (12): 1247-64.

Lunn, W., S. Pasiakos, M. Colletto, K. Karfonta, J. Carbone, J. Anderson, and N. Rodriguez. 2012. "Chocolate Milk and Endurance Exercise Recovery: Protein Balance, Glycogen and Performance." *Medicine & Science in Sports & Exercise* 44 (4): 682-91.

MacDonald, G., D. Button, E. Drinkwater, and D. Behm. 2014. "Foam Rolling as a Recovery Tool After an Intense Bout of Physical Activity." *Medicine & Science in Sports & Exercise* 46 (1): 131-42.

MacDonald, G., M. Penney, M. Mullaley, A. Cuconato, C. Drake, D. Behm, and D. Button. 2013. "An Acute Bout of Self-Myofascial Release Increases Range of Motion Without a Subsequent Decrease in Muscle Activation or Force." *Journal of Strength and Conditioning Research* 27 (3): 812-21.

MacKenney, M., K. Miller, J. Deal, J. Garden-Robinson, and Y. Rhee. 2015. "Plasma and Electrolyte Changes in Exercising Humans After Ingestion of Multiple Boluses of Pickle Juice." *Journal of Athletic Training* 50 (2): 141-46.

McDermott, B., S. Anderson, L. Armstrong, D. Casa, S. Cheuvront, L. Cooper, L. Kenney, F. O'Connor, and W. Robert. 2017. "National Athletic Trainers' Association Position Statement: Fluid Replacement for the Physically Active." *Journal of Athletic Training* 52 (9): 877-95.

Miller, K., G. Mack, and K. Knight. 2009. "Electrolyte and Plasma Changes After Ingestion of Pickle Juice, Water and a Common Carbohydrate-Electrolyte Solution." *Journal of Athletic Training* 44 (5): 454-61.

Peake, J., O. Neubauer, N. Walsh, and R. Simpson. 2017. "Recovery of the Immune System After Exercise." *Journal of Applied Physiology* 122: 1077-87.

Pritchett, K., R. Pritchett, and P. Bishop. 2012. "Nutritional Strategies for Post-Exercise Recovery: A Review." *South African Journal of Sports Medicine* 23 (1): 20. https://doi.org/10.17159/2078-516x/2011/v23ila370.

Suni, E. 2022. "How Sleep Works: Understanding the Science of Sleep." Sleep Foundation. Updated October 19, 2022. www.sleepfoundation.org/how-sleep-works.

Weinberg, C. 2016. "Can Cupping Really Speed Post-Workout Recovery?" Vocativ.com. Accessed December 17, 2018. www.vocativ.com/news/350152/cupping-recovery/index.html.

Chapter 7

Hausswirth, C., and I. Mujika. 2013. *Recovery for Performance in Sport.* Champaign, IL: Human Kinetics.

MacDonald, G.Z., M.D.H. Penney, M.E. Mullaley, A.L. Cuconato, C.D.J. Drake, D.G. Behm, and D.C. Button. 2013. "An Acute Bout of Self-Myofascial Release Increases Range of Motion Without a Subsequent Decrease in Muscle Activation or Force." *Journal of Strength and Conditioning Research* 27 (3): 812-21.

Verkoshansky, Y., and M. Siff. 2009. *Supertraining.* 6th ed. Denver, CO: Supertraining Institute.

Chapter 8

Bompa, T., and C. Buzzichelli. 2015. *Periodization Training for Sports.* 3rd ed. Champaign, IL: Human Kinetics.

Haff, G.G., and N.T. Triplett. 2016. *Essentials of Strength Training and Conditioning.* 4th ed. Champaign, IL: Human Kinetics.

Hausswirth, C., and I. Mujika. 2013. *Recovery for Performance in Sport.* Champaign, IL: Human Kinetics.

Schoenfeld, B. 2021. *Science and Development of Muscle Hypertrophy.* 2nd ed. Champaign, IL: Human Kinetics.

Verkoshansky, Y., and M. Siff. 2009. *Supertraining.* 6th ed. Denver, CO: Supertraining Institute.

Zatsiorsky, V., W. Kraemer, and A.C. Fry. 2020. *Science and Practice of Strength Training.* 3rd ed. Champaign, IL: Human Kinetics.

Chapter 9

Arent, S., H. Cintineo, B. McFadden, A. Chandler, and M. Arent. 2020. "Nutrient Timing: Garage Door of Opportunity?" *Nutrients* 12 (7): 1948-67.

Bushman, B. 2013. "Exercise and Sleep." *ACSM's Health & Fitness Journal* 17 (5): 5-8.

Chennaoui, M., P. Arnal, F. Sauvet, and D. Leger. 2014. "Sleep and Exercise: A Reciprocal Issue?" *Sleep Medicine Reviews* 20: 59-72.

French, D., and L. Ronda. 2022. *NSCA's Essentials of Sport Science.* Champaign, IL: Human Kinetics.

Gladding, R. 2013. "This Is Your Brain on Meditation." *Psychology Today,* May 22, 2013. www.psychologytoday.com/us/blog/use-your-mind-change-your-brain/201305/is-your-brain-meditation.

Haff, G.G., and N.T. Triplett. 2016. *Essentials of Strength Training and Conditioning.* 4th ed. Champaign, IL: Human Kinetics.

Kenney, W., J. Wilmore, and D. Costill. 2022. *Physiology of Sport and Exercise.* 8th ed. Champaign, IL: Human Kinetics.

Kersick, C., S. Arent, B. Schoenfeld, J. Stout, B. Campbell, C. Wilborn, L. Taylor, et al. 2017. "International Society of Sports Nutrition Position Stand: Nutrient Timing." *Journal of the International Society of Sports Nutrition* 14: 33.

McCall, P. 2018. "Why Meditation Should Be a Part of Your Fitness Routine." *24Life.com.* Accessed March 2023. www.24life.com/why-meditation-should-be-a-part-of-your-fitness-routine.

Meier, U., and A. Gressner. 2004. "Endocrine Regulation of Energy Metabolism: Review of Pathobiochemical and Clinical Chemical Aspects of Leptin, Ghrelin, Adiponectin, and Resistin." *Clinical Chemistry* 50 (9): 1511-25.

Mifflin, M.D., S.T. St. Jeor, L.A. Hill, B.J. Scott, S.A. Daugherty, and Y.O. Koh. 1990. "A New Predictive Equation for Resting Energy Expenditure in Healthy Individuals." *American Journal of Clinical Nutrition* 51 (2): 241-47.

Sedlmeier, J., J. Eberth, M. Schwarz, D. Zimmermann, F. Haarig, S. Jaeger, and S. Kunze. 2012. "The Psychological Effects of Meditation: A Meta-Analysis." *Psychological Bulletin* 138 (6): 1139-71.

Suni, E. 2022. "How Sleep Works: Understanding the Science of Sleep." Sleep Foundation. Updated October 19, 2022. www.sleepfoundation.org/how-sleep-works.

Thomas, D.T, K.A. Erdman, and L.M. Burke. 2016. "American College of Sports Medicine Joint Position Statement. Nutrition and Athletic Performance." *Medicine & Science in Sports & Exercise* 48 (3): 543-68.

Valley Health System. 2017. "What Is Mindfulness-Based Meditation and Why Should I Try It?" *ScienceDaily.com,* June 19, 2017. www.sciencedaily.com/releases/2017/06/170619134340.htm.

INDEX

ABOUT THE AUTHOR

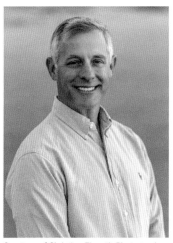

Courtesy of Christine Ekeroth Photography.

Pete McCall is the director of education for EōS Fitness, the host of the *All About Fitness* podcast, a strength coach, and a fitness educator. He is certified as a personal trainer through the American Council on Exercise (ACE) and the National Academy of Sports Medicine (NASM), and he holds a CSCS (Certified Strength and Conditioning Specialist) certification from the National Strength and Conditioning Association (NSCA).

Frequently quoted as a fitness expert in publications such as the *Washington Post, Wall Street Journal, U-T San Diego Union Tribune, Time, Men's Fitness, SELF, Glamour, U.S. News & World Report,* and *Shape* magazine, McCall is a sought-after resource for accurate, in-depth insight into how to get results from exercise. Besides working with individual clients and teaching group fitness classes, he has more than a decade of experience in educating personal trainers around the world, including teaching for both ACE and NASM.

McCall is a former exercise physiologist for ACE, where he helped create the Integrated Fitness Training (ACE IFT) model, write the *ACE Personal Trainer Manual,* and develop education workshops on metabolic conditioning, movement-based training, and youth fitness. He is a master trainer for Core Health & Fitness (the parent company of Nautilus, StairMaster, Star Trac, and Schwinn), a content contributor for 24 Hour Fitness, and an adjunct faculty member in exercise science at both Mesa Community College and San Diego State University. He has delivered wellness education talks for the U.S. Navy (at Naval Air Station North Island), the White House, the World Bank, the International Association of Fire Fighters, and Reebok.

McCall earned his master's of science degree in exercise science and health promotion from the California University of Pennsylvania, and he holds the Fellow in Applied Functional Science credential from the Gray Institute.

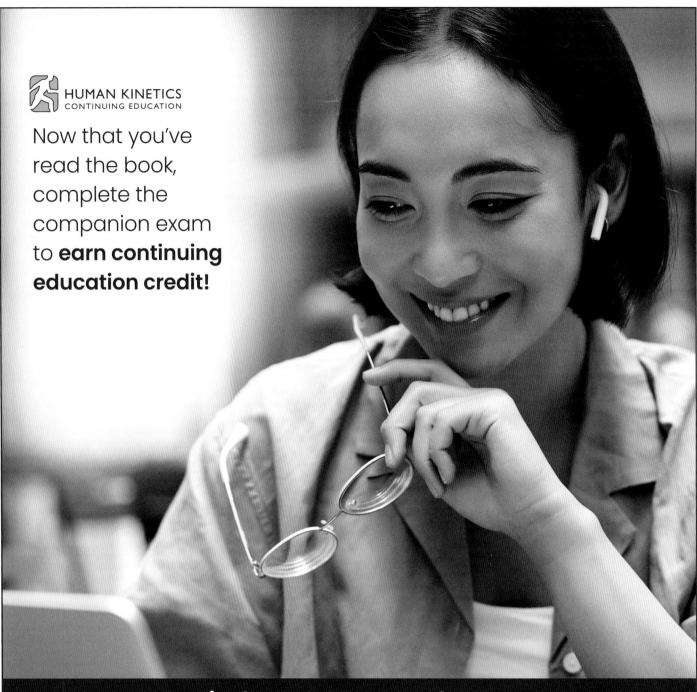